CONGENITAL HEART DISEASE

CONGENITAL HEART DISEASE

A Deductive Approach to Its Diagnosis

BURTON W. FINK, M.D.

Director, Pediatric Cardiology, Cedars-Sinai Medical Center, Los Angeles, California; *Clinical Professor,* Pediatrics (Cardiology), University of California, Los Angeles

YEAR BOOK MEDICAL PUBLISHERS, INC.
Chicago • London

Library of Congress Catalog Card Number: 74-83117

International Standard Book Number: 0-8151-3222-0

Reprinted, May 1977

*To Janet, Susan and Elaine, for whom the future is;
and to Flo, with whom my future will be*

Foreword

IF SOMEONE were to ask me whether there is a need today for another textbook on pediatric cardiology, I would say "No." But this book is different, and I urged Doctor Fink to tackle the job when he first mentioned the thought of writing it.

Almost 30 years ago, when I first became interested in pediatric cardiology, there were almost no comprehensive sources of information on the subject. Since then, the field has had its golden age and a number of excellent comprehensive textbooks have appeared that fully document the accumulated knowledge and experience. In addition, there are other books involving specific subareas of pediatric cardiology.

The beginning student of congenital heart disease has a problem today when so much is to be learned in finding a source that will efficiently provide him with the knowledge he needs. This book will make his task easier.

The author is an outstanding teacher. His effectiveness stems from a deep interest in students and a native ability that I have long admired and envied. His success is evident, because regularly each year he is given the Outstanding Teacher Award by his House Staff. He has developed a technique of instruction employing mnemonics and his own style of language. The student is guided to an understanding of congenital heart disease by logic and reasoning rather than by rote. As a result, the learning experience is smooth and retention of information is considerably enhanced.

Doctor Fink mercifully has first narrowed the field for the harassed beginning student by choosing the most common congenital cardiac anomalies and presenting only the basics, i.e., embryology, anatomy, hemodynamics, clinical picture and differential diagnosis. Second, he has presented the subject material in his own special style.

The result, I believe, is a valuable contribution to the beginning student of congenital heart disease and to the established physician who wishes to refresh his knowledge on the subject or add to it. He or she will find this volume easy to read, an excellent learning source and, therefore, highly rewarding for the time spent.

SAMUEL O. SAPIN

Preface

FOR THE PAST 17 years I have had the privilege of teaching pediatric cardiology to medical students and house officers. I have long believed that the techniques that have been successfully employed in teaching by lecture and seminar would be equally effective in teaching by the printed word. This concept was the stimulus for this book. By designing the book primarily for the physician in training, I have taken certain liberties: it is short; each chapter is self-contained; treatment has been omitted; the language is less technical than it is literary; certain knowledge is presumed or not expected and certain data are idealized.

I believe if a person can envision the anatomic malformations that result from errors in embryologic development, a deductive approach to the diagnosis of congenital heart disease can be utilized. Thus, each chapter begins with the embryology and anatomy. A mnemonic then follows that links the anatomy and physiology in a diagrammatic line drawing from which the hemodynamics are developed and the clinical findings are evolved. The chapter ends with a differential diagnosis and a group of "pearls," which, by my definition, are items to which deduction cannot always logically be applied.

The book, therefore, in a very real sense, is as much one of method as it is one of facts. As such, it does not pretend to be either a definitive treatise or a reference volume. These types of texts are readily available and are listed in the bibliography.

It is hoped that because of the composition, size and teaching method employed, the physician in practice as well as the physician in training will find the book an easy reference for a brief review of an immediate problem.

ACKNOWLEDGMENTS

I wish to thank, beyond words, Dr. Samuel Sapin, who reviewed every word and every diagram for clarity and accuracy. Without his aid, my task would have been immeasurably more difficult and the end product less valuable.

I would thank Trus. J. Thies, who supervised the reproduction work, and Gary Marshall and Martin Fong, who worked with her. A very special compliment must be extended to Lydia Wisniewski, who carefully and meticulously executed the original art work. The photographs and illustrations were done in the Department of Audio-Visual Services of the Cedars-Sinai Medical Center in Los Angeles, California.

The patience and accuracy of Grace Johnson, my personal secretary, in doing the final typing and collating are deeply appreciated.

And, last, an expression of gratitude to each of the medical students and house officers whom I have had the privilege of teaching. For through their stimulation and intellectual challenge, I have grown.

BURTON W. FINK

Table of Contents

CHAPTER ONE
Atrial Septal Defect

EMBRYOLOGY

FROM APPROXIMATELY the fourth to the sixth week of gestation, the single atrial chamber is effectively divided into two. This is begun by the growth of a thin wall of tissue — the first septum — which originates in the dorsal wall of the single atrium and proceeds in its growth toward the endocardial cushions. These are concomitantly growing to separate the atria from the ventricles. As the first septum approaches these cushions, the space between the two structures is called the ostium primum, or first hole (Fig. 1–1, A). As it proliferates to seal totally, fenestrations appear in the center of the first septum, leading to a second hole — the ostium secundum. At this time there appears a second thin septum growing to the right of the first — the septum secun-

Fig. 1–1.—Schematic representation of the formation of the interatrial septum. **A**, 30 days; **B**, 33 days; **C**, 37 days; **D**, newborn. (See text for explanation.) (Modified from Moss, A. J., and Adams, F. H. [eds.]: *Heart Disease in Infants, Children and Adolescents* [Baltimore: The Williams & Wilkins Company, 1968], p. 16.)

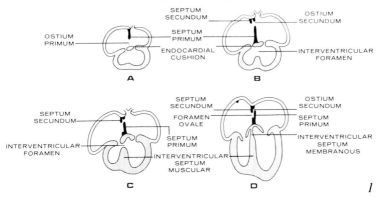

1

dum (Fig. 1–1, *B*). The ultimate balance between proliferation and absorption in these two septa leads to the formation of a hole – the foramen ovale – to be guarded on its left side by a valve (Fig. 1–1, *C* and *D*). This arrangement effectively permits blood flow from the right atrium to the left atrium during fetal development. After birth, when left atrial pressure exceeds right atrial pressure, flow in either direction is prevented.

ANATOMY

If there is an error in this development in either the amount of material laid down or the amount of material reabsorbed, a communication will result between the two atria, which is termed an atrial septal defect. If the interatrial communication is high in the septum near the junction of the superior vena cava and the right atrium, and if one of the right pulmonary veins

Fig. 1–2. – Schematic representation of the various types of atrial septal defect. **A**, sinus venosus, **B**, Chiari network, **C**, ostium secundum, **D**, ostium primum.

drains anomalously into that site, it is entitled a sinus venosus defect. Should there be multiple fenestrations of the central portion of the septum, it is called a Chiari network. If the hole is in the center of the septum, it is known as an ostium secundum defect. If the communication is at the location of the ostium primum — the lower end of the septum — it is logically called an ostium primum defect. (The latter usually is accompanied by a defect in the mitral valve and can be classified as an incomplete atrioventricular canal or a partial endocardial cushion defect.) (Fig. 1 – 2.)

HEMODYNAMICS

The patient with an atrial septal defect has a burden placed on the right side of his heart as a result of an increase in volume — enormous at times — coursing through the atrial septum from the left atrium to the right atrium. This is conceptualized in the mnemonic

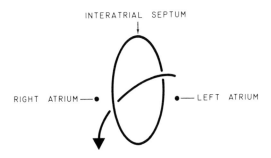

The arrow represents blood flowing from the left atrium through the interatrial septum into the right atrium. If the flow of blood is followed with the mnemonic in mind, the effect on the size of the various components of the heart can be demonstrated by the following diagram:

RIGHT ATRIUM ↑	LEFT ATRIUM →
RIGHT VENTRICLE ↑	LEFT VENTRICLE →
MAIN PULMONARY ARTERY ↑	AORTA → ↓
PULMONARY VESSELS ↑	

Fig. 1–3.—Chest roentgenograms of a patient with an atrial septal defect. Note the cardiomegaly, enlargement of the right atrium, right ventricle, pulmonary artery and apparent decrease in the aorta. The pulmonary markings are increased. RA = right atrium, RV = right ventricle, PA = pulmonary artery, Ao = aorta, PV = pulmonary vessels.

Fig. 1–4.—Electrocardiogram of a patient with an ostium secundum type of atrial septal defect. The salient features are a dominant S_1 and R_{III}, which is right axis deviation, and the rSR′ in V_1 and prominent $SV_{5, 6}$, which are interpretable as right ventricular hypertrophy.

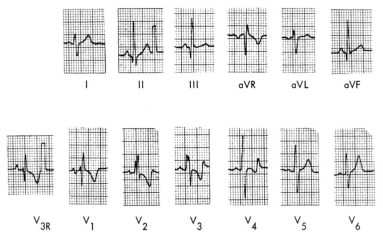

The arrows represent alteration in the size of a chamber or a vessel as follows:

$\rightarrow$ Unchanged
$\uparrow$ Increased
$\downarrow$ Decreased

This information can logically be translated to the chest x-ray, where one would predict an enlarged right atrium, right ventricle, main pulmonary artery, an increase in the vascular markings of the lungs and a relatively normal left side. Such is the case as seen in Figure 1 – 3. Although there are basic changes in volume, these are reflected in the electrocardiogram as a form of mild right ventricular hypertrophy (Fig. 1 – 4).

CLINICAL APPLICATION

The increased volume of blood presented to the right ventricle is ejected through the pulmonary valve in ventricular systole. This creates the typical ejection murmur, usually grade II/VI in intensity, which can be heard at the second left interspace and transmits along the course of the pulmonary vessels. This same volume of blood had passed through the tricuspid valve during atrial systole (ventricular diastole), leading to the frequently heard mid-diastolic filling sound in the area of the fourth or fifth interspace to the left of the sternum. The fixed overload of the right ventricle results in a prolonged ejection time of that chamber and consistently delays the closure of the pulmonary valve. This results in a wide splitting of the second sound. With expiration, venous return normally is decreased, but due to the fixed volume overload of the shunt, right ventricular ejection is not altered significantly. Thus, the second sound will retain its fixed splitting, being unaffected by respiration.

The patient with this lesion characteristically is asymptomatic. The appearance of the murmur will draw attention to its presence. The diagnosis can clinically be suspected in such a patient who may be slightly smaller in structure, who is functioning normally, has a prominent left chest, an ejection systolic mur-

TABLE 1–1.—IDEALIZED CARDIAC CATHETERIZATION DATA
IN A PATIENT WITH AN ATRIAL SEPTAL DEFECT*

SITE	PRESSURE (mm Hg)		OXYGEN SATURATION (%)	
	Normal	Patient	Normal	Patient
Superior vena cava			70	72
Inferior vena cava			74	76
Right atrium	a = 5 v = 3 m = 4	a = 5 v = 3 m = 4	72	85
Right ventricle	25/2	40/2	72	85
Main pulmonary artery	25/12	30/12	72	85
Right pulmonary artery	25/12	30/12	72	85
Systemic artery	120/80	120/80	97	97
Left atrium	a = 5 v = 7 m = 6	a = 4 v = 5 m = 4	97	97

*The salient features are an increase in oxygen saturation at the level of the right atrium, a slight increase in right ventricular pressures with a slight gradient across the pulmonary valve and similar mean pressures in both the right and left atria.

mur at the second left interspace, a fixed widely split second sound and perhaps a diastolic filling sound at the lower left sternal border. Suspicion would be intensified if the chest x-ray was abnormal as described and the electrocardiogram showed right ventricular hypertrophy. The diagnosis can be confirmed by heart catheterization, during which an increase in oxygen saturation in the right atrium and equal pressure in the two atria would be found (Table 1–1).

OSTIUM PRIMUM DEFECT

The patient with an ostium primum type defect has all of the same physiologic challenges as one with an ostium secundum defect. In addition, because of the cleft in the mitral valve, mitral insufficiency is present also. This combination of events can cause poor growth and development and congestive heart failure in infancy. The diagnosis can be suspected in a patient who has all the signs and symptoms of an atrial septal defect as discussed

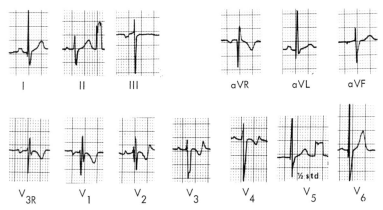

Fig. 1—5.—Electrocardiogram of a patient with an ostium primum type of atrial septal defect. The salient features are a dominant R_1 and S_{III}, which is left axis deviation, and the rSR′ in V_1 and prominent $SV_{5, 6}$, which are interpretable as right ventricular hypertrophy.

but who has left axis deviation in the electrocardiogram (Fig. 1–5). Cardiac catheterization will be similar to that in a patient with an ostium secundum defect, with the additional finding of an abnormal mitral valve as demonstrated by angiocardiography.

DIFFERENTIAL DIAGNOSIS

The patient with an atrial septal defect must be differentiated from one having moderate pulmonary stenosis or an innocent murmur.

The murmur of mild pulmonary stenosis is similar but usually somewhat harsher and has with it a variably split second sound and frequently a diminished pulmonary component of that sound. The vascular markings, as seen on the chest x-ray, should be normal. Cardiac catheterization may be necessary to differentiate the two.

The patient with an innocent murmur will also have a second sound that is entirely normal. In addition, the murmur will vary considerably with changes in position and with exercise.

PEARLS

1. Atrial septal defect occurs more commonly in females than in males.

2. The patients are, in the main, asymptomatic.

3. It is extraordinarily rare to have patients become symptomatic in early infancy.

4. Patients with atrial septal defect rarely go into heart failure.

5. The development of marked pulmonary hypertension with reversal of shunt flow is a late phenomenon and is very rare in the pediatric age range.

6. Right ventricular pressures in the catheterization laboratory in excess of 50 millimeters of mercury strongly suggest a coexisting complicating lesion.

7. Because of rapid flow, mixing of the shunt may be demonstrated in the right ventricle rather than the right atrium. This could lead to an erroneous diagnosis of a ventricular septal defect. Clinical correlation is needed.

8. Atrial septal defect is seen commonly with the Holt-Oram syndrome.

9. If the diagnosis of atrial septal defect is suspected and the electrocardiogram shows left axis deviation, an ostium primum defect must be seriously considered.

CHAPTER TWO
Ventricular
Septal Defect

EMBRYOLOGY

BETWEEN the fourth and eighth weeks of gestation, the single ventricular chamber is effectively divided into two. This is accomplished by fusion of the membranous portion of the ventricular septum, the endocardial cushions and the bulbus cordis (the proximal portion of the truncus arteriosus). The muscular portion of the ventricular septum grows cephalad as each ventricular chamber enlarges, eventually meeting with the right and left ridges of the bulbus cordis. The right ridge fuses with the tricuspid valve and the endocardial cushion, thus separating the pul-

Fig. 2−1.−Schematic representation of the formation of the interventricular septum. **A,** 30 days; **B,** 33 days; **C,** 37 days; **D,** newborn. (See text for explanation.) (Modified from Moss, A. J., and Adams, F. H. [eds.]: *Heart Disease in Infants, Children and Adolescents* [Baltimore: The Williams & Wilkins Company, 1968], p. 16.)

Fig. 2−2.−Schematic representation of the role of the bulbus cordis in the formation of the interventricular septum. (See text for explanation.)

monary valve from the tricuspid valve. The left ridge fuses with a ridge of the interventricular septum, leaving the aortic ring in continuity with the mitral ring. The endocardial cushions are concomitantly developing and ultimately fuse with the bulbar ridges and the muscular portion of the septum. The final closure and separation of the two ventricles is made by the fibrous tissue of the membranous portion of the interventricular septum (Figs. 2 – 1 and 2 – 2).

ANATOMY

Failure of adequate development of any of the component parts, namely, the muscular portion of the interventricular septum, the endocardial cushions or the bulbar ridges (truncoconal ridges) will result in a communication between the two ventricles —a ventricular septal defect. The defect between the two ventricles may lie above the crista supraventricularis, beneath the pulmonary valve, below the crista supraventricularis in the membranous septum or below the crista supraventricularis in the muscular septum. The particular relationship between the membranous portion of the septum and the floor of the right atrium makes possible a direct communication between these two chambers. This permits an anatomic classification of ventricular septal defect into those above the crista supraventricularis, those below the crista supraventricularis and those in direct communication between the left ventricle and the right atrium.

HEMODYNAMICS

Initially, the patient with a ventricular septal defect could be considered as merely having a communication between the left and the right ventricle, with shunt flow generally going from left to right. But a ventricular septal defect is not a simple lesion, for between the two ventricles sits the pulmonary vascular bed, which not only is influenced by the lesion itself but may exert its own independent influence on the lesion. To better understand this lesion, as well as patent ductus arteriosus and others, the various changes that take place in the pulmonary arterioles and their effect on pulmonary resistance need to be elaborated. Three different courses can be anticipated.

First, at the time of delivery and with the first breath, the lungs expand and the pulmonary arterioles dilate. There follows gradual resolution of the fetal musculature of the arterioles, with a drop in resistance occurring over several days to several months. The vessels finally reach their adult character, with a large lumen, thin intima and reasonable musculature. These findings may remain unaltered despite the presence of a left-to-right shunt.

Second, after normal involution, the arterioles, in the presence of a persistent left-to-right shunt at the ventricular level, are the recipients of increased flow under an increased head of pressure, which may alter the pulmonary vessels by mechanical means, chemical means, or both. The vessels respond with hypertrophy of the muscular layer followed by thickening of the intimal layer, which, individually or in combination, can cause elevation of the pulmonary resistance.

Third, in some patients, for reasons that as yet are not clear, the fetal vasculature fails to mature and the high initial pulmonary resistance remains elevated independent of any cardiac defect.

The intertwining of the location and size of ventricular septal defects and pulmonary vascular resistance is such that it would be wise to consider each variation individually.

CLASSIC VENTRICULAR SEPTAL DEFECT

Hemodynamics

This defect can be conceptualized in the mnemonic

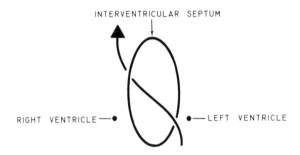

The arrow represents blood flowing from the left ventricle through the interventricular septum into the right ventricle and out the pulmonary artery. If the flow of blood is followed with the mnemonic in mind, the effect on the various chambers and vessels of the heart can be demonstrated by the following diagram:

RIGHT ATRIUM →	LEFT ATRIUM ↑
RIGHT VENTRICLE → ↑	LEFT VENTRICLE ↑
MAIN PULMONARY ARTERY ↑	AORTA →
PULMONARY VESSELS ↑	

The arrows represent alteration in the size of a chamber or a vessel as follows:

→ Unchanged
↑ Increased

Translated to the chest x-ray, there would be possible enlargement of the right ventricle, definite enlargement of the main pulmonary artery, an increase in the pulmonary vessels and en-

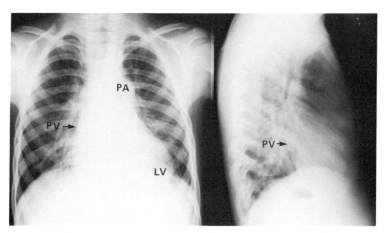

Fig. 2–3.—Chest roentgenograms of a patient with a classic ventricular septal defect. Note the cardiomegaly, enlargement of the left ventricle and the increase in the pulmonary artery. The left atrium is not clearly seen. The pulmonary markings are increased. *LV* = left ventricle, *PA* = pulmonary artery, *PV* = pulmonary vessels.

Fig. 2–4.—Electrocardiogram of a patient with a classic ventricular septal defect. The salient features are a dominant R wave in V_1 and a dominant R wave in $V_{5, 6}$, which are interpretable as combined ventricular hypertrophy.

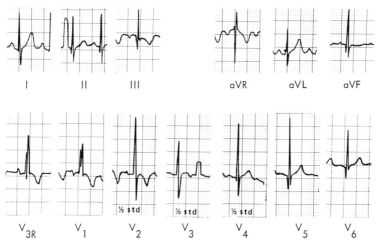

largement of the left atrium and left ventricle (Fig. 2–3). The electrocardiogram will vary from left ventricular hypertrophy (not shown) to combined ventricular hypertrophy (Fig. 2–4).

Clinical Application

With the onset of left ventricular contraction, blood flows immediately through the ventricular defect into the right ventricle, lasting throughout all of systole and giving rise to a holosystolic murmur. It is heard best at the fourth interspace to the left of the sternum, and will have widespread transmission throughout most of the anterior chest and even into the area of the pulmonary artery. It may be heard in the back by direct transmission. The shunted blood returns to the left atrium and may create a murmur in diastole as it flows through the mitral valve. This would be heard at the apex. The systolic murmur usually is of such intensity (grade IV/VI) as to create a palpable thrill. The increased right-sided volume may delay closure of the pulmonary valves. Since the right ventricle will be influenced by venous return in addition to the shunt flow, the closure of the pulmonary valve will vary with respirations. The intensity of the closure of

TABLE 2–1.–IDEALIZED CARDIAC CATHETERIZATION DATA IN A CHILD WITH A CLASSIC VENTRICULAR SEPTAL DEFECT*

SITE	PRESSURE (mm Hg)		OXYGEN SATURATION (%)	
	Normal	Patient	Normal	Patient
Superior vena cava			70	70
Inferior vena cava			74	74
Right atrium	a=5 v=3 m=4	a=5 v=3 m=4	72	72
Right ventricle	25/2	40/4	72	85
Main pulmonary artery	25/12	40/14	72	85
Left atrium	a=5 v=7 m=6	a=5 v=7 m=6	97	97
Systemic artery	120/80	120/80	97	97

*The salient features are an increase in oxygen saturation at the level of the right ventricle and slightly elevated pressures in the right ventricle and the main pulmonary artery.

the pulmonary valves will vary directly with the degree of pulmonary hypertension present. The activity of the left ventricle will be reflected by a palpable thrust, felt laterally on the chest. If there is significant right ventricular enlargement, this will be demonstrated by a palpable heave to the left of the sternum. Cardiac catheterization will demonstrate an increase in oxygen saturation at the level of the right ventricle and minimally elevated pressures in the right ventricle and main pulmonary artery (Table 2 – 1).

SMALL VENTRICULAR SEPTAL DEFECT

Hemodynamics

The mnemonic shown previously is applicable to this physiologic state as well. However, because of diminished blood flow, the effect on the chambers of the heart will be negligible and can be represented in the following diagram:

RIGHT ATRIUM →	LEFT ATRIUM →
RIGHT VENTRICLE →	LEFT VENTRICLE →
PULMONARY ARTERY →	AORTA →
LUNGS →	

Since the alterations in chamber and vessels are negligible, it is predictable that both the chest x-ray and the electrocardiogram would be normal. This is indeed the case and they are not demonstrated.

Clinical Application

One variety of this size of defect is Roger's ventricular septal defect. The classic holosystolic murmur located at the fourth interspace to the left of the sternum accompanied by a palpable thrill and a normal second sound would be expected. It must be emphasized, however, that other very small ventricular septal defects have their own clinical profile. In these, the flow through the defect occurs with the onset of systole but stops in the middle of systole, when muscular contraction of the septum may occlude the hole. This would give rise to a much softer (grade II/VI) early to midsystolic murmur localized to the fourth and fifth left interspace without significant transmission. The second sound would remain normal. Cardiac catheterization would show a very small increase in oxygen saturation at the level of the right ventricle. Indicator dilution techniques often are required to confirm the lesion. However, most patients in this group are diagnosed clinically and handled medically without catheterization.

SUPRACRISTAL VENTRICULAR SEPTAL DEFECT

The peculiar location of this defect above the crista supraventricularis permits flow from the left ventricle almost directly into the pulmonary artery. Keeping in mind the location of such flow, one might expect that the murmur, also holosystolic in nature, would be higher in the chest at the first and second interspace to the left of the sternum, with transmission occasionally into the neck. This usually is not the case. The murmur most often is very much like that heard in a classic defect. A thrill would accompany the murmur. The second sound would vary as that in a classic variety. The chest x-ray, electrocardiogram and catheterization would be similar to those of the classic defect. This variety most commonly is found as a surprise at surgery, recognized as being in an unusual location by the surgeon.

EISENMENGER'S COMPLEX

By definition, this is a clinical situation wherein a patient with a ventricular septal defect (or any other left-to-right shunt for that matter) has developed sufficient pulmonary vascular disease and pulmonary hypertension to cause the shunt through the defect to become right to left.

Hemodynamics

The concept is demonstrated in the two mnemonics

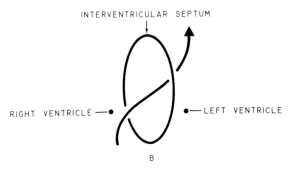

Remembering the definition of Eisenmenger's complex, the effect on the heart is demonstrated in *A*. When conditions worsen, mnemonic *B* applies. The effect on the chambers and vessels can be demonstrated in the following diagram:

RIGHT ATRIUM ↑
RIGHT VENTRICLE ↑
PULMONARY ARTERY ↑
LUNGS ↑ ↓

LEFT ATRIUM ↑ →
LEFT VENTRICLE → ↑
AORTA → ↑

Applied to the chest x-ray, one would expect to find an enlarged right atrium and right ventricle, an enlarged pulmonary artery, prominent proximal and small distal pulmonary vessels and a left atrium and left ventricle varying in size (Fig. 2–5). The electrocardiogram would demonstrate the dominant right ventricular hypertrophy (Fig. 2–6).

Fig. 2–5.—Chest roentgenograms of a patient with Eisenmenger's complex. Note the gross cardiomegaly and increase in size of the right atrium, right ventricle and pulmonary artery. The proximal pulmonary vessels are dilated whereas the distal vessels are normal in size. *RA* = right atrium, *RV* = right ventricle, *PA* = pulmonary artery, *PV* = pulmonary vessels.

Clinical Application

The generalized cardiomegaly will cause a prominence of the left side of the chest and a displacement of the apical impulse laterally and downward. Enlargement of the right ventricle will be recognized by a palpable heave along the left sternal border and enlargement of the left ventricle by a palpable thrust at the apex. The development of pulmonary hypertension has caused the right ventricular pressure to increase to the level of the systemic pressure. There being no gradient between the two ventricles, no shunting would take place and therefore no murmur will be heard. As the shunting diminishes, right ventricular ejection time shortens, permitting the pulmonary valve to close sooner. As pulmonary hypertension increases, the intensity of the pulmonary valve closure will increase also. Therefore, with Eisen-

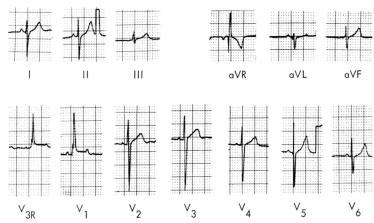

Fig. 2–6.—Electrocardiogram of a patient with Eisenmenger s complex. The salient features are the dominant S_I and R_{III}—right axis deviation. There also is a dominant R wave in V_1 and S wave in $V_{5, 6}$, which is interpretable as right ventricular hypertrophy. The T wave in V_1 is also upright.

TABLE 2–2.—IDEALIZED CARDIAC CATHETERIZATION DATA
IN A CHILD WITH AN EISENMENGER COMPLEX*

SITE	PRESSURE (mm Hg)		OXYGEN SATURATION (%)	
	Normal	Patient	Normal	Patient
Superior vena cava			70	62
Inferior vena cava			74	66
Right atrium	a = 5 v = 3 m = 4	a = 11 v = 7 m = 6	72	64
Right ventricle	25/2	120/4	72	64
Main pulmonary artery	25/12	120/80	72	64
Right pulmonary artery	25/12	120/80	72	64
Systemic artery	120/80	120/80	97	92–82†
Left atrium	a = 5 v = 7 m = 6	a = 8 v = 10 m = 7	97	97

*The salient features are generalized decreased oxygen saturations in the right side of the heart with no increase at the level of the right ventricle. The systemic artery has a slightly decreased oxygen saturation at rest and a significantly decreased value (†) when stressed. In addition, the pressures in the right ventricle and the pulmonary artery are systemic in height.

menger's complex, one can anticipate a very narrowly split second sound, with significant increase in the intensity of the pulmonary component. With time and progression of the disease process, pulmonary resistance exceeds systemic resistance and the shunt through the ventricular septal defect reverses, resulting in systemic cyanosis. Cardiac catheterization will demonstrate peripheral arterial desaturation and right ventricular and pulmonary arterial pressures that equal systemic values (Table 2–2).

LEFT VENTRICLE TO RIGHT ATRIAL SHUNT

Hemodynamics

This very special variety of ventricular septal defect can be depicted in the mnemonic

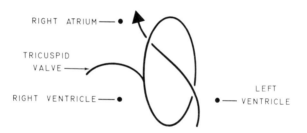

The arrow represents blood flowing from the left ventricle directly into the right atrium.

The effect of this blood flow can be shown in the following diagram:

RIGHT ATRIUM ↑	LEFT ATRIUM ↑
RIGHT VENTRICLE ↑	LEFT VENTRICLE ↑
PULMONARY ARTERY ↑	AORTA → ↑
LUNGS ↑	

Applied to the chest x-ray, one would expect to find an enlargement of the right atrium, right ventricle, pulmonary artery and lung fields. The left atrium may be enlarged also, as would the left ventricle. The electrocardiogram would show combined ventricular hypertrophy and possibly right atrial hypertrophy and would resemble that seen in an atrial septal defect. These are not demonstrated.

Clinical Application

The similarity between this variety of ventricular septal defect and the ostium secundum type of atrial septal defect should be apparent. The chest might be more prominent on the right side, with a right ventricular heave, but a left ventricular thrust might be present also. The flow going from a high-pressure chamber to a low-pressure chamber would more likely resemble the holosystolic murmur of the classic ventricular septal defect. It would, however, be somewhat higher in the chest and would be accompanied by a thrill. The second sound would reflect the constant overload of the right ventricle and would more closely approximate that of the atrial septal defect. A wide split would be anticipated and variability with respiration would be minimal. Cardiac catheterization would be useful to define the lesion where one would expect an increase in oxygen saturation at the level of the right atrium. Left ventricular angiography would show the communication between that chamber and the right atrium.

NATURAL HISTORY OF VENTRICULAR SEPTAL DEFECT

The information presented to this point now can be utilized to present an over-all view of this anatomic entity and its variations, thereby giving a portrait of its natural history.

The newborn has virtually equal resistances in both the pulmonary and systemic circuits. The patient with a ventricular septal defect will be no different. His pressures in the right and left ventricles will be equal also and no murmur can be expected to be present at birth. As the resistance in the lungs falls, there is a concomitant drop in the right ventricular pressure, creating a gradient between the two ventricles. The flow then can take place and a murmur will be heard. The initial physiologic effect of the increased flow is to burden the left atrium and ventricle with an increased volume. If this occurs gradually, accommodation is possible and no clinical problem will result. If, however, the volume burden is acute and overwhelming, heart failure will ensue.

One patient may be born normally, present with the appearance of a murmur at 2 – 6 weeks of age, be totally asymptomatic and grow in a normal fashion, keeping his defect but apparently unaffected by it. Another patient may be born normally, present with a murmur at 2 – 6 weeks of age, be totally asymptomatic, grow in a normal fashion but by 1 year of age have the murmur disappear. This is believed to represent spontaneous closure of the ventricular septal defect and may occur in as high as 10 – 30% of patients. Another patient may be born normally, present with the appearance of a murmur at 2 – 6 weeks of age and prove to have a clinically significant defect. With time, however, and through a mechanism not clearly understood, hypertrophy of the right ventricular infundibulum takes place. This patient will improve clinically, for the flow into the pulmonary circuit will be diminished. Another patient may be born normally, present with a murmur at 2 – 6 weeks of age and at that time, or shortly thereafter, go into heart failure. At catheterization, very large shunt flows will be present along with low pulmonary resistance (remember that resistance equals pressure divided by flow). These patients, when compensated, will grow but usually poorly. Some can be maintained to an age suitable for elective repair whereas others will remain in such congestive failure that an early surgical approach will be required. A last group of patients will be born apparently normal, present with a murmur at 2 – 6 weeks of age but grow poorly, although not necessarily suffer congestive heart failure. When catheterized, they will be found to have pulmonary resistances approaching systemic levels, with moderate to minimal left-to-right shunts.

The troublesome fact is that it is impossible to predict which course an infant with a ventricular septal defect will take. Therefore, it becomes necessary at this time to use serial catheterizations in an attempt to ascertain the course that the patient is following.

DIFFERENTIAL DIAGNOSIS

The patient with a ventricular septal defect must be differentiated from a patient with idiopathic hypertrophic subaortic stenosis, a patent ductus arteriosus, an atrial septal defect, an innocent murmur and noncyanotic tetralogy of Fallot.

The patient with idiopathic hypertrophic subaortic stenosis has a murmur that varies in intensity, occurs later in systole and is altered significantly by venous return and is mentioned in the differential only because the location of the murmur is at the same general location as that of the ventricular septal defect.

The patient with an atrial septal defect is only momentarily confused with one having a left ventricle to right atrial type of ventricular septal defect. The absence of a thrill and the much quieter murmur should help make the differential. Cardiac catheterization should permit an accurate differentiation.

Although the innocent murmur of the "twangy string" variety is heard at the same general location, it is early and mid in systole, lower in pitch and very variable in its characteristics. In addition, the patient will have a normal chest x-ray and electrocardiogram.

If the patient with a ventricular septal defect develops secondary infundibular hypertrophy, he then will resemble the patient with noncyanotic tetralogy of Fallot. If the patient has been followed clinically, the appearance of a decreased pulmonary component of the second sound in the presence of right ventricular hypertrophy on the electrocardiogram will suggest the presence of acquired infundibular stenosis. If, however, such a clinical course is not known, a differentiation may not be possible.

In infancy, the patient with a patent ductus arteriosus generally only has a systolic murmur that may be indistinguishable from that heard in a patient with a ventricular septal defect. Cardiac catheterization will be required to effect the differential.

PEARLS

1. Ventricular septal defect occurs more commonly in males than in females.

2. *The murmurs heard in early infancy, which disappear by 1 year of age, probably represent defects that have closed spontaneously.*

3. *Some patients maintain elevated pulmonary resistances despite therapy directed at the ventricular septal defect and may, in fact, represent a primary disease of the pulmonary vessels.*

4. *In infancy, a ventricular septal defect may be indistinguishable from a patent ductus arteriosus.*

5. *The axiom "The louder the murmur the smaller the defect" does not always apply.*

CHAPTER THREE

Patent Ductus Arteriosus

EMBRYOLOGY

BETWEEN the fifth and seventh weeks of gestation, the aortic arch system develops (Fig. 3–1). This begins as six paired arches proliferating from the apex of the truncus arteriosus. The sixth, or pulmonary, arch gives off a branch that grows toward the developing lung. On the right side, the proximal portion becomes the proximal portion of the right pulmonary artery and the distal portion disappears. On the left side, the proximal portion becomes the proximal portion of the left pulmonary artery but the distal portion maintains its attachment to the aorta, becoming the ductus arteriosus.

Fig. 3–1.—Diagrammatic representation of the development of the aortic arch system as it relates to the ductus arteriosus. Note that the left pulmonary artery and the ductus arteriosus were the embryonic sixth arch.

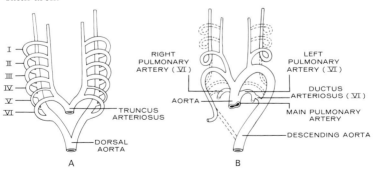

25

ANATOMY

During fetal life, the ductus arteriosus serves as a functioning connection between the pulmonary artery and the aorta. After birth and with institution of respiration, the Po_2 rises and the pulmonary arterioles dilate, each of which influences the ductus arteriosus to close. Ultimately, it will fibrose, becoming the ligamentum arteriosum. Under certain circumstances, however, the vessel remains open, being called, somewhat redundantly, a patent ductus arteriosus.

HEMODYNAMICS

The patient with a patent ductus arteriosus has an abnormal communication between the aorta with its high pressure and the pulmonary artery with its low pressure, through which a volume of blood flows. This places a volume burden on the lungs and ultimately on the left side of the heart, a situation not dissimilar to the patient with a ventricular septal defect. This is conceptualized in the mnemonic

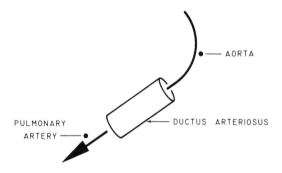

The arrow represents blood flowing from the aorta through the ductus arteriosus into the pulmonary artery. It is also meant to represent the circumstances present in the older infant and young child after the pulmonary vessels have matured and before any supervening secondary pulmonary hypertension has developed. If the flow is followed, its effect on the heart can be demonstrated by the following diagram:

RIGHT ATRIUM →	LEFT ATRIUM → ↑
RIGHT VENTRICLE →	LEFT VENTRICLE → ↑
MAIN PULMONARY ARTERY ↑	AORTA ↑
PULMONARY VESSELS ↑	

The arrows represent alteration in the size of a chamber or a vessel as follows:

→ Unchanged
↑ Increased

Translated to the chest x-ray, the pulmonary artery, pulmonary vessels and the aorta would rather consistently be increased in size. The size of the left atrium and left ventricle would be variable, depending on the magnitude of the shunt (Fig. 3–2). If pulmonary hypertension were present, the right ventricle would be enlarged also.

The electrocardiogram would be equally variable, ranging

Fig. 3–2.—Chest roentgenograms of a 7-year-old patient with patent ductus arteriosus. The salient features are the absence of a significant cardiomegaly, the presence of a full pulmonary artery segment, a prominent aortic knob and increased pulmonary vessels. Note that on the lateral view the left ventricle is not significantly enlarged. *PA* = pulmonary artery, *Ao* = aorta, *PV* = pulmonary vessels, *LV* = left ventricle.

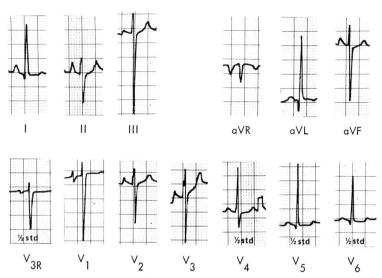

Fig. 3–3.—Electrocardiogram of a 7-year-old patient with patent ductus arteriosus showing left ventricular hypertrophy. The salient features are a deep S wave in V_1 and a tall R wave in V_5. In addition, the axis deviation of the bipolar leads is leftward.

from a normal tracing (not shown) to left ventricular hypertrophy (Fig. 3–3) or combined ventricular hypertrophy (Fig. 3–4). In the face of pulmonary hypertension, right ventricular hypertrophy would be seen (not demonstrated).

CLINICAL APPLICATION

The patient with a patent ductus arteriosus is influenced by changes in the pulmonary vascular bed quite like the patient with a ventricular septal defect. The reader is referred to Chapter 2 for a detailed explanation. It is usual at birth for the resistances in both pulmonary and systemic circuits to be identical. As normal resolution of the pulmonary arterioles takes place, the pulmonary resistance falls, the pulmonary artery pressure drops and a gradient is created between the aorta and the pulmonary artery. Flow then can take place across the ductus. It is

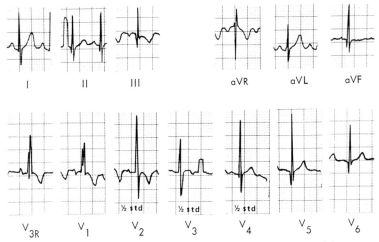

I   II   III   aVR   aVL   aVF

V$_{3R}$ V$_1$ V$_2$ V$_3$ V$_4$ V$_5$ V$_6$

½ std   ½ std   ½ std

Fig. 3–4. — Electrocardiogram of a 6-year-old patient with patent ductus arteriosus showing combined ventricular hypertrophy. The salient features are a dominant R wave in V$_1$, a dominant R wave in V$_5$ and V$_6$ and tall complexes in V$_{2, 3, 4}$.

common in this age range for there to be a wide pulse pressure in the arterial system, but the diastolic pressure in both the pulmonary artery and the aorta are virtually identical (Fig. 3–5). Flow through the ductus then would take place only during systole and therefore only a systolic murmur would be heard. By

Fig. 3–5. — A representative pullback pressure curve in a patient with a patent ductus arteriosus. Note that the diastolic pressure in the aorta and the main pulmonary artery are identical. The systolic pressure in the ventricle is the same as that in the pulmonary artery. *Ao* = aorta, *MPA* = main pulmonary artery, *RV* = right ventricle.

Ao 92/32   MPA 64/32   RV 60/4

the latter half of the first year, with continued maturation in both systemic and pulmonary vessels, a diastolic gradient will also develop, flow will take place in both systole and diastole and the classic continuous murmur will be heard. The murmurs will occur to the left of the sternum at the second and third inter-spaces and will transmit not only down the sternum anteriorly but along the course of the pulmonary arteries, being heard quite well in the back. The volume of blood presented to the left side of the heart will cause displacement of the apex laterally and inferiorly. A left ventricular thrust usually will be felt. Increased left ventricular volume may prolong the systolic ejection time, thereby delaying closure of the aortic valve. The right side of the heart will be affected by variations of venous return and there-fore a normal splitting of the second sound can be anticipated. The intensity of closure of the pulmonary valve will depend on the pulmonary artery pressure and the pulmonary resistances. If the patient is not treated and if pulmonary hypertension devel-ops, the pulmonary valve will close with greater intensity and somewhat earlier than normal, creating narrowing of the splitting sound with an intensification of the pulmonary component.

TABLE 3–1.—IDEALIZED CARDIAC CATHETERIZATION DATA IN A 2-MONTH-OLD PATIENT WITH A PATENT DUCTUS ARTERIOSUS*

SITE	PRESSURE (mm Hg)		OXYGEN SATURATION (%)	
	Normal	Patient	Normal	Patient
Superior vena cava			70	70
Inferior vena cava			74	74
Right atrium	a = 5 v = 4 m = 4	a = 5 v = 4 m = 4	72	72
Right ventricle	25/2	60/5	72	72
Main pulmonary artery	25/12	60/30	72	84
Left atrium	a = 5 v = 7 m = 6	a = 7 v = 9 m = 8	97	97
Left ventricle	90/5	90/5	97	97
Systemic artery	90/50	90/30	97	97

*The salient features are an increase in oxygen saturation in the pulmonary artery, elevation of the systolic pressure in the pulmonary artery and equal diastolic pressures in the pulmonary artery and the systemic artery. The pressure in the left atrium is slightly elevated also.

Extrapolation of this information to the patient now can be attempted. The patient with a patent ductus arteriosus usually will be considered normal at birth. No murmur will be reported. By 2–6 weeks of age, flow may begin through the ductus and a systolic murmur will be heard. The left atrium and ventricle will

Fig. 3–6.—An enlarged photograph of a 35-mm cineangiocardiographic frame, showing the classic course of a cardiac catheter in a patient with a patent ductus arteriosus. Note the passage of the catheter from the right side of the heart through the ductus arteriosus into the descending aorta. *RA* = right atrium, *RV* = right ventricle, *MPA* = main pulmonary artery, *DA* = ductus arteriosus, *Ao* = descending aorta, *C* = catheter.

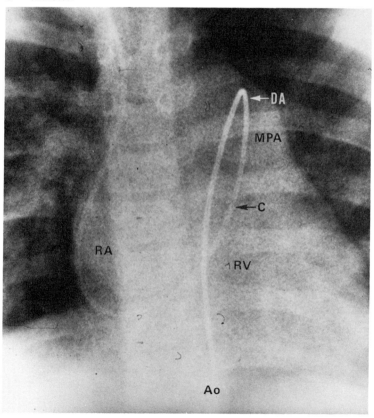

become recipients of a considerable volume overload, leading to two possible courses: First, if the left ventricle cannot accommodate to the load, an increase in diastolic pressure will occur, leading to an increase in left atrial pressure and pulmonary venous engorgement. The patient may develop a cough, dyspnea, tachypnea and tachycardia, followed by hepatosplenomegaly — the classic symptoms and signs of congestive heart failure. This infant with a patent ductus arteriosus may be indistinguishable from one with a ventricular septal defect, and cardiac catheterization most often is needed to establish an accurate diagnosis. It will show an increase in oxygen saturation at the level of the pulmonary artery, thus differentiating it from a ventricular septal defect. In addition, the systolic pressure in the pulmonary artery will be elevated but less than that in the systemic artery whereas the diastolic pressure in each will be virtually the same (Table 3–1). Passage of the catheter through the ductus arteriosus into the descending aorta will make the diagnosis absolute (Fig. 3–6). Second, if the left ventricle can accommodate to the load, the infant remains asymptomatic and the presence of congenital heart disease is announced merely by the appearance of a systolic murmur. The patient's growth pattern may be reasonable, and ultimately the appearance of a typical continuous murmur permits a clinical diagnosis of a patent ductus arteriosus, obviating the absolute need for catheterization.

DIFFERENTIAL DIAGNOSIS

The patient with a patent ductus arteriosus must be distinguished from one having a venous hum, a pulmonary arteriovenous fistula, a coronary arteriovenous fistula, a sinus of Valsalva aneurysm and stenoses of the pulmonary arteries.

Differentiation from the venous hum is most important, for the latter is an innocent phenomenon relating to venous return. It is heard most commonly over the second right interspace but can be present over the second left interspace when a left superior vena cava is present. The murmur tends to disappear with compression of the neck vessels, turning of the head or assumption of a supine position, each of which alters the quantity and quality of venous return. It is notable that a venous hum virtually always disappears when the patient is lying down whereas the murmur of a patent ductus arteriosus remains or frequently increases with lying down.

A pulmonary arteriovenous fistula has a comparable continuous murmur but it usually is heard over lung tissue some distance from the heart. If it were present in vessels overlying the heart, further confusion would exist and cardiac catheterization might be needed to effect the diagnosis.

The murmur of a coronary arteriovenous fistula resembles that of the patent ductus but is heard lower on the chest and has a greater diastolic accentuation. Cardiac catheterization, however, almost always will be required to confirm this diagnosis.

The murmur of a sinus of Valsalva aneurysm may be very reminiscent of a patent ductus arteriosus and would require cardiac catheterization for definition.

Stenoses of the pulmonary arteries also may have a continuous murmur but the diastolic phase frequently is inconsistent. The murmur usually is heard under both clavicles, with transmission through the pulmonary vessels equally to the right and left. Cardiac catheterization may be necessary to differentiate it from a patent ductus arteriosus. (This lesion is discussed in greater detail in Chapter 6.)

PEARLS

1. Patent ductus arteriosus occurs more commonly in females than in males.

2. In the infant, bounding posterior tibial and dorsalis pedis pulses help to differentiate a patent ductus arteriosus from a ventricular septal defect.

3. A classic continuous murmur in the first months of life should make one consider other diagnoses before a patent ductus arteriosus.

4. In the premature infant, normal closure of the ductus arteriosus may be delayed beyond the newborn period.

5. The disappearance of the continuous murmur in the supine position supports the diagnosis of a venous hum and is against the diagnosis of a patent ductus arteriosus.

CHAPTER FOUR

Endocardial Cushion Defect

EMBRYOLOGY

BETWEEN the fourth and eighth weeks of gestation, the transition from a tubular heart into a four-chambered structure is completed. This is accomplished through four events, namely, septation at the level of the atria (Fig. 4–1), septation at the level of the ventricles (Fig. 4–1), proliferation of the endocardial cushions (Fig. 4–2) and growth of the bulboconus area (Fig. 4–3). The single atrium is divided by growth of a thin wall of tissue — the first septum — which originates in the dorsal wall of the

Fig. 4–1. — Schematic representation of the formation of the interatrial and interventricular septum. **A,** 30 days; **B,** 33 days; **C,** 37 days; **D,** newborn period. (See text for explanation.) (Modified from Moss, A. J., and Adams, F. H. [eds.]: *Heart Disease in Infants, Children and Adolescents* [Baltimore: The Williams & Wilkins Company, 1968], p. 16.)

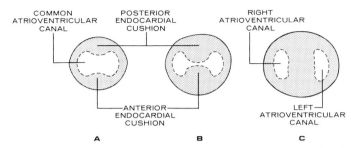

Fig. 4–2. – Schematic representation in cross section showing how the endocardial cushions divide the common atrial ventricular canal into two. (See text for explanation.)

single atrium and proceeds in its growth toward the endocardial cushions. These are concomitantly growing to separate the atria from the ventricles. As the first septum approaches these cushions, the space between the two structures is called the ostium primum or first hole (see Fig. 4–1, *A*). As it proliferates to seal totally, fenestrations appear in the center of the first septum, leading to a second hole – the ostium secundum. At this time there appears a second thin septum growing to the right of the first – the septum secundum (see Fig. 4–1, *B*). The ultimate balance between proliferation and absorption in these two septa leads to the formation of a hole – the foramen ovale – to be

Fig. 4–3. – Schematic representation of the role of the bulbus cordis in the formation of the interventricular septum. (See text for explanation).

guarded on its left side by a valve (see Fig. 4–1, *C* and *D*). This arrangement effectively permits blood flow from the right atrium to the left atrium during fetal development. After birth, when left atrial pressure exceeds right atrial pressure, flow in either direction is prevented.

Between the fourth and eighth weeks of gestation, the single ventricle is divided by fusion of the membranous portion of the ventricular septum, the endocardial cushions and the bulbus cordis (the proximal portion of the truncus arteriosus). The muscular portion of the ventricular septum grows cephalad as each ventricular chamber enlarges, eventually meeting with the right and left ridges of the bulbus cordis. The right ridge fuses with the tricuspid valve and the endocardial cushion, thus separating the pulmonary valve from the tricuspid valve. The left ridge fuses with a ridge of the interventricular septum, leaving the aortic ring in continuity with the mitral ring. The endocardial cushions (see Fig. 4–2) are concomitantly developing and ultimately fuse with the bulbar ridges (see Fig. 4–3) and the muscular portion of the septum. The final closure and separation of the two ventricles is made by the fibrous tissue of the membranous portion of the interventricular septum (see Fig. 4–1).

ANATOMY

If the endocardial cushions do not fuse, the atrioventricular valves – tricuspid and mitral – cannot develop properly. In addition, the lower portion of the interatrial septum and the upper portion of the interventricular septum will be deficient and will be unable to meet with the endocardial cushions. This will result in a large central hole and free communication among all four chambers – the complete form of an endocardial cushion defect (Fig. 4–4). Endocardial cushion defects have been classified as partial, transitional and complete. The first is an ostium primum defect and is discussed in Chapter 1. The transitional form has partial fusion of the endocardial cushions, resulting in variable abnormalities of the atrioventricular valves, and is not discussed. It is the purpose of this chapter to deal only with the complete form.

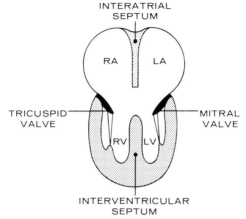

Fig. 4–4.—Schematic representation of the anatomy in a complete endocardial cushion defect. The salient feature is a large central hole. (See text for explanation.) *RA* = right atrium, *RV* = right ventricle, *LA* = left atrium, *LV* = left ventricle.

HEMODYNAMICS

The patient with an endocardial cushion defect has the potential for blood flow between any of the four chambers of the heart. This flow is dependent on the relative resistances of the pulmonary and systemic circuits, the pressures within the two ventricular chambers and the relative compliance of all the chambers. This concept is shown in the mnemonic

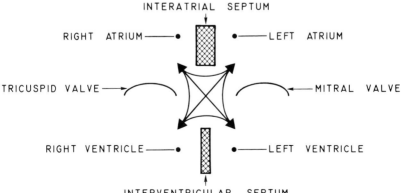

If the blood is followed with the mnemonic in mind, the effect on the various chambers and vessels of the heart can be demonstrated by the following diagram:

RIGHT ATRIUM ↑	LEFT ATRIUM ↑
RIGHT VENTRICLE ↑	LEFT VENTRICLE ↑
MAIN PULMONARY ARTERY ↑	AORTA →
PULMONARY VESSELS ↑	

The arrows represent alteration in the size of a chamber or a vessel as follows:

→Unchanged

↑ Increased

This information can be translated to the chest x-ray, where one would expect to find gross cardiomegaly, enlargement of all four chambers and increased vascular markings (Fig. 4–5). The electrocardiogram also shows combined ventricular hypertrophy and possibly combined atrial hypertrophy. The frontal-plane QRS forces would be directed in a counterclockwise fashion, with the intial deflection being rightward and then leftward and

Fig. 4–5.—Chest roentgenograms of a patient with an endocardial cushion defect. Note the gross cardiomegaly, with enlargement of all four intercardiac chambers. The pulmonary vessels are increased. *RA* = right atrium, *RV* = right ventricle, *LA* = left atrium, *LV* = left ventricle, *PV* = pulmonary vessels.

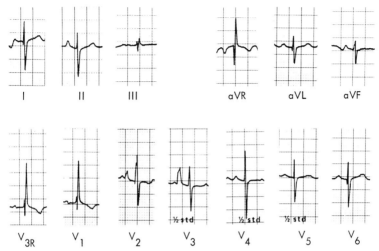

Fig. 4–6.—Electrocardiogram of a patient with an endocardial cushion defect. The salient features are a Q wave in leads I and aVL and a deep S wave in lead aVF, which is interpretable as left axis deviation with a counterclockwise inscription of the QRS forces. There also is a tall R' in lead V_1, a deep S in lead V_6 and tall complexes in leads $V_{3, 4, 5}$, which are interpretable as combined ventricular hypertrophy.

superiorly, producing left axis deviation as expressed by the presence of a Q wave in leads I and aVL and a deep S wave in lead aVF (Fig. 4–6).

CLINICAL APPLICATION

It has been suggested that at this point there is potential flow between any of the cardiac chambers at any one time. In addition, pulmonary hypertension of a marked degree is rather consistently present. These two facts influence the clinical picture. Growth is poor, respiratory infections are common and congestive heart failure is frequent. The gross cardiomegaly will cause a prominent left chest and the specific chamber enlargement will be responsible for a right ventricular heave and a left ventricular thrust. In the presence of pulmonary hypertension, intensified closure of the pulmonary valve will be palpable as a tap high on the left side of the chest. All peripheral pulses will be palpable and not unusual. The presence of mitral and tricuspid insufficiency, atrial septal defect and a ventricular septal defect would prompt one to anticipate murmurs representing any or all of these phenomena. This may indeed be the case, but quite often the clinical situation is one of balanced intracardiac dynamics and minimal abnormal shunting, resulting in virtually no murmurs. The presence of pulmonary hypertension is heralded by a single or closely duplicated second sound, with the pulmonary component being significantly increased in intensity. (The latter is the auscultatory equivalent of the pulmonary closure tap.)

The patient may be suspected of having a complete endocardial cushion defect if he has poor growth and development, a prominent left chest, variable murmurs or none at all, an increased pulmonary component of the second sound, gross cardiomegaly on chest x-ray with increased vascular markings and an electrocardiogram with an abnormal leftward axis and biven-

TABLE 4–1.—IDEALIZED CARDIAC CATHETERIZATION DATA IN AN INFANT WITH AN ENDOCARDIAL CUSHION DEFECT*

SITE	PRESSURE (mm Hg)		OXYGEN SATURATION (%)	
	Normal	Patient	Normal	Patient
Superior vena cava			70	65
Inferior vena cava			74	70
Right atrium	a = 5 v = 3 m = 4	a = 10 v = 10 m = 9	72	75
Right ventricle	25/2	100/7	72	80
Main pulmonary artery	25/12	100/50	72	80
Pulmonary vein	a = 6 v = 8 m = 7	a = 8 v = 10 m = 9	97	97
Left atrium	a = 5 v = 7 m = 6	a = 8 v = 10 m = 8	97	86
Left ventricle	100/5	100/5	97	82
Systemic artery	100/75	100/75	97	82

*The salient features are an increase in oxygen saturation at the right atrium, a further increase at the right ventricle, a decrease in oxygen saturation at the left atrium and a further decrease at the level of the left ventricle. The pressures in the right ventricle and the pulmonary artery are systemic in height whereas those in each atrium are slightly elevated.

tricular hypertrophy. The diagnosis can be confirmed with cardiac catheterization, which would show the ability to pass the catheter into all four chambers but in a bizarre manner, such as from the right atrium directly to the left ventricle, bidirectional intracardiac shunting and systemic pressures in the right ventricle and pulmonary artery (Table 4–1).

DIFFERENTIAL DIAGNOSIS

The patient with a complete endocardial cushion defect must be differentiated from one having pulmonary hypertension with any other lesion. This would include such lesions as a ventricular septal defect with pulmonary hypertension (the Eisenmenger complex), an ostium primum type of an atrial septal defect, a patent ductus arteriosus in an infant and a type I, II, III truncus arteriosus. The electrocardiogram will be of major help in making the correct diagnosis. It should be commented that on occasion a patient with a ventricular septal defect will have an electrocardiogram with left axis deviation, which will be confusing; in this circumstance, cardiac catheterization will be necessary to effect the differential.

PEARLS

1. The complete form of endocardial cushion defect is the most common cardiac anomaly seen in patients with Down's syndrome.

2. Early and unremitting pulmonary hypertension is the rule.

3. There is no sex preference for the lesion.

CHAPTER FIVE

Aortic Stenosis and Other Lesions Obstructive to Left Ventricular Outflow

EMBRYOLOGY

BETWEEN the sixth and ninth weeks of gestation, the truncus arteriosus is divided into the aorta and the pulmonary artery. At about the same time, the aortic valves develop. These are formed by proliferation of three tubercles within the lumen of the aorta, which grow toward the midline (Fig. 5–1). Where the tubercle joins the wall of the aorta there is resorption of tissue

Fig. 5–1.—Demonstration of formation of the aortic valves within the aorta. Note the progressive proliferation of the truncoconal ridges. (The pulmonary valves are also demonstrated coincidentally.) (Modified from Moss, A. J., and Adams, F. H. [eds.]: *Heart Disease in Infants, Children and Adolescents* [Baltimore: The Williams & Wilkins Company, 1968], p. 16.)

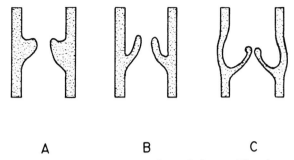

A   B   C

Fig. 5–2. – A graphic representation of the proliferation and then hollowing out of the tubercles, giving rise to the completed valve.

Fig. 5–3. – Diagrammatic representation of the various types of obstruction to left ventricular outflow. **A,** discrete subvalvular stenosis, **B,** idiopathic hypertrophic subaortic stenosis, **C,** valvular aortic stenosis, **D,** supravalvular aortic stenosis. LV = left ventricle, •→ = site of obstruction.

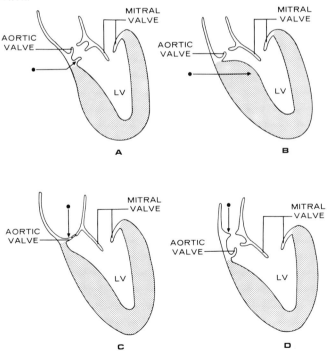

followed by further hollowing out of tissue, giving rise to the sinuses of the valve (Fig. 5–2). During the seventh week of gestation, the coronary arteries develop.

ANATOMY

Obstruction to left ventricular outflow can occur below the valve in either a fixed discrete or variable muscular form, at the valve itself or above the valve (Fig. 5–3). Although similarities exist among the anatomic varieties, the differences are sufficient to warrant a separate discussion of each. The most common variation will be discussed first.

VALVULAR AORTIC STENOSIS

Hemodynamics

The patient with valvular aortic stenosis has an obstruction to left ventricular ejection at the level of the valve, which is demonstrated in the mnemonic

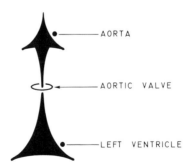

The arrow represents blood flowing from the left ventricle through the obstructed aortic valve into the aorta. The thickened base of the arrow, labeled left ventricle, is meant to represent the increased pressure required to overcome the resistance of the obstructed valve. The head of the arrow represents blood in the ascending aorta. The size of the head is meant to suggest dissipation of energy into the vessel itself. If the blood flow is followed with the mnemonic in mind, the effect on the heart can be demonstrated by the following diagram:

RIGHT ATRIUM →	LEFT ATRIUM →
RIGHT VENTRICLE →	LEFT VENTRICLE ↑
MAIN PULMONARY ARTERY →	ASCENDING AORTA ↑
PULMONARY VESSELS →	

The arrows represent alteration in the size of a chamber or a vessel as follows:

→ Unchanged
↑ Increased

This information can be translated to the chest x-ray, where the right side of the heart will be normal, the left ventricle enlarged and the ascending aorta dilated. Since the effect of the obstruction on the left ventricle is one of muscular hypertrophy rather than dilatation, the over-all size of the heart generally is not increased (Fig. 5–4). The electrocardiogram will show left ventricular hypertrophy (Fig. 5–5).

Clinical Application

If the patient survives infancy without challenge, he generally will grow without difficulty and appear to be normal. The selective hypertrophy of the left ventricle displaces the apex laterally and inferiorly, which can be seen and also felt as a thrust. The first sound will be normal. On opening, the impaired mobility of the aortic valves will cause them to vibrate against the wall of the aorta and will be recognized as an ejection click. Since the aortic valves are located at about the fourth interspace to the left of the sternum, that is where the click will be heard. The murmur follows immediately afterward, is systolic in time, ejection in nature, low-pitched and harsh in quality and varying in intensity from grade II/VI to grade VI/VI. Even though the murmur is generated as blood passes through the aortic valve, it is heard best at the second interspace to the right of the sternum—the location of maximal intensity of the transmitted sound. Once the intensity reaches or exceeds grade IV/VI, a palpable thrill will accompany the murmur, being present both at the second right interspace and in the suprasternal notch. The thickened nature

Fig. 5–4.—Chest roentgenograms of a child with valvular aortic stenosis. Note the slightly dilated ascending aorta and the left ventricular enlargement. *LV* = left ventricle, *Ao* = aorta.

Fig. 5–5.—Electrocardiogram of a patient with valvular aortic stenosis. The salient features are the deep S wave in V_1 and tall R waves in $V_{5, 6}$, which are interpretable as left ventricular hypertrophy.

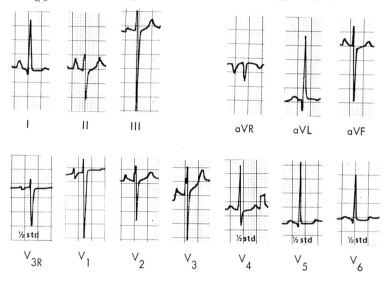

of the stenotic valve will cause it to close with a less than normal intensity, resulting in a diminished aortic component of the second sound. The more severe the stenosis the greater will be the ejection time of the left ventricle and the later will the aortic valve close. This will result in a narrowing of the splitting of the second sound. If the stenosis is extraordinarily severe, the aortic valve will, in fact, close after the pulmonary valve and will be recognized as a reversed splitting of the second sound. (This can be identified either clinically or with a phonocardiogram by a narrowing of the splitting with inspiration and a widening of the splitting with expiration.) The intracardiac events will be reflected in the peripheral arterial pulse, which will have a prolonged upstroke with an anacrotic notch, a single sustained peak and a slow downstroke (Fig. 5–6, *C*). The systemic arterial pressure will have a diminished peak systolic value and a narrow pulse

Fig. 5–6.—Diagrammatic representation of the various types of peripheral arterial pulse curves in the various forms of obstruction to left ventricular outflow. **A,** normal, **B,** idiopathic hypertrophic subaortic stenosis, **C,** valvular aortic stenosis, **D,** supravalvular aortic stenosis, with *RA* being the right arm and *LA* being left arm. *AN* = anacrotic notch, *SP* = systolic peak, *DN* = dicrotic notch. (See text for explanation.)

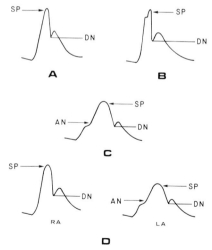

pressure. When the aortic stenosis is due to abnormalities of a three-leaflet valve, aortic insufficiency is uncommon. When the valve is bicuspid in nature, aortic insufficiency frequently is present and is recognized by the presence of a high-pitched decrescendo diastolic murmur along the left sternal border.

The diagnosis of valvular aortic stenosis can be suspected in a patient—generally a male—who has a small peripheral pulse with a delayed upstroke, a narrow pulse pressure, a left ventricular thrust, a systolic ejection click followed by a systolic ejection murmur and a palpable thrill at the second right interspace or in the suprasternal notch. The chest x-ray would show left ventricular enlargement and a dilated ascending aorta. The electrocardiogram would show left ventricular hypertrophy. The diagnosis can be confirmed with cardiac catheterization, during which one would find an elevated left ventricular systolic pressure with a diminished aortic systolic pressure, the gradient occurring at the valve. Oxygen saturations will be normal (Table 5–1). Cineangiocardiography will demonstrate the nature of the obstructed valve.

If the aortic valve is very severely stenosed, the challenge to the patient is immediate and presents its own unique clinical pic-

TABLE 5–1.—IDEALIZED CARDIAC CATHETERIZATION DATA
IN A CHILD WITH VALVULAR AORTIC STENOSIS*

SITE	PRESSURE (mm Hg)		OXYGEN SATURATION (%)	
	Normal	Patient	Normal	Patient
Superior vena cava			70	70
Inferior vena cava			74	74
Right atrium	a = 5 v = 4 m = 4	a = 5 v = 4 m = 4	72	72
Right ventricle	25/2	25/2	72	72
Main pulmonary artery	25/12	25/12	72	72
Left ventricle	110/5	160/10	97	97
Aorta	110/80	90/70	97	97

*The salient features are elevated pressures in the left ventricle and diminished pressures with a narrow pulse pressure in the aorta. The oxygen saturations are normal.

ture. The infant — usually a male — will be in heart failure, with the classic signs of tachypnea, tachycardia and hepatomegaly. It must be remembered that the anatomic location of the aortic valve is at about the fourth interspace to the left of the sternum. In the infant, the murmur generated by turbulent flow through the stenotic orifice is not only generated at but often is heard best at that location. As such, it may be confused with the murmur caused by flow through a ventricular septal defect.

IDIOPATHIC HYPERTROPHIC SUBAORTIC STENOSIS

Hemodynamics

The obstruction to left ventricular outflow is related to the asymmetric enlargement of the left side of the ventricular septum and the proximity of the anterior leaflet of the mitral valve to that septal hypertrophy. It must be clearly understood that this lesion is a dynamic one and that the obstruction is variable, which results in physical findings that are equally variable. The concept of the obstruction is demonstrated in the mnemonic

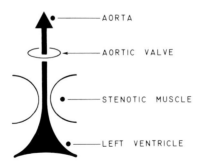

The arrow represents blood flowing from the left ventricle past the obstructive muscle through a normal aortic valve into the aorta. The thickened base of the arrow represents the increased pressure required to overcome the resistance offered by the stenotic muscle. The head of the arrow represents the blood in the aorta and is not enlarged, suggesting the absence of extraordinary pressure in that vessel. If the blood flow is followed with the mnemonic in mind, the effect on the heart can be shown in the following diagram:

RIGHT ATRIUM →	LEFT ATRIUM → ↑
RIGHT VENTRICLE →	LEFT VENTRICLE ↑
MAIN PULMONARY ARTERY →	ASCENDING AORTA →
PULMONARY VESSELS →	

The arrows are meant to represent alteration in a chamber or vessel as follows:

→ Unchanged
↑ Increased

This information can be translated to the chest x-ray, where the right side of the heart will be normal, the left ventricle enlarged, but the ascending aorta will not be dilated. There generally is cardiomegaly (Fig. 5–7). The electrocardiogram will show varying degrees of left ventricular hypertrophy and Figure 5–5 will be representative.

Clinical Application

It must be emphasized that the area of obstruction is subvalvular and that the valves themselves are normal. As the left ventricle enlarges, the apex will be displaced laterally and inferiorly and will be visible and also felt as a thrust. With systolic contraction, the obstruction is met and a midsystolic ejection murmur results. Because the obstruction is below the valve, this murmur generally is heard near the apex. Occasionally, transmission of the murmur into the ascending aorta may take place and be heard at the second interspace to the right of the sternum but it rarely transmits into the neck vessels. If the murmur is of sufficient intensity, a thrill will accompany it and be felt near the apex. The aortic valves being normal, an ejection click generally is not heard, the second sound is normal and aortic insufficiency is not present.

The dynamic nature of this entity is further demonstrated by the variability of the findings when the patient is challenged with certain physiologic modalities. Amyl nitrite, which decreases

Fig. 5–7.—Chest roentgenograms of a child with idiopathic hypertrophic subaortic stenosis. Note the cardiac enlargement with specific left ventricular enlargement and the absence of dilatation of the ascending aorta. *LV* = left ventricle, *Ao* = aorta.

systemic blood pressure, and the Valsalva maneuver, which decreases venous return, each increases the gradient and thereby increases the intensity of the murmur. Contrariwise, a nonpharmacologic event, such as clenching of the fists or squatting, elevates systemic blood pressure, decreases the gradient and causes a diminution of the murmur.

The systolic events are translated into an unusual peripheral pulse curve, in which there is an immediate initial rapid upstroke followed by a second upstroke shortly thereafter. The pulse pressure tends to be normal (see Fig. 5–6, *B*).

The diagnosis of idiopathic hypertrophic subaortic stenosis can be suspected in a patient—generally an adolescent male—who has a rapid upstroke of his arterial pulse, a left ventricular thrust, the absence of a systolic ejection click but the presence of a systolic ejection murmur, loudest near the apex with virtually no transmission into the neck and which increases in intensity with the Valsalva maneuver and decreases in intensity with clenching of the fists or squatting. The chest x-ray would show cardiomegaly with left ventricular enlargement and the electrocardiogram would show left ventricular hypertrophy. Echocardi-

TABLE 5-2.—IDEALIZED CARDIAC CATHETERIZATION DATA IN A CHILD WITH IDIOPATHIC HYPERTROPHIC SUBAORTIC STENOSIS*

SITE	PRESSURE (mm Hg)		OXYGEN SATURATION (%)	
	Normal	Patient	Normal	Patient
Superior vena cava			70	70
Inferior vena cava			74	74
Right atrium	a = 5 v = 4 m = 5	a = 5 v = 4 m = 5	72	72
Right ventricle	25/2	25/2	72	72
Main pulmonary artery	25/12	25/12	72	72
Left ventricle	110/5	170/7	97	97
Left ventricle — subvalvular	110/5	110/5	97	97
Aorta	110/80	110/75	97	97

*The salient features are an increase in pressure in the left ventricle and a decrease in pressure in the subvalvular area of the left ventricle and the aorta. The oxygen saturations are normal.

ography may demonstrate the apposition of the anterior leaflet of the mitral valve to the left side of the ventricular septum. Confirmation can be obtained with cardiac catheterization, during which one finds elevated left ventricular pressure near the apex but diminished left ventricular pressure in the subvalvular area and in the ascending aorta (Table 5–2). Cineangiocardiography will demonstrate the abnormality of the left ventricular outflow tract.

DISCRETE SUBVALVULAR STENOSIS

The fibrous ring with the narrowed central orifice that sits just below the normal aortic valves results in physical findings that are quite similar to those seen in valvular aortic stenosis. The chest is symmetric. With enlargement of the left ventricle, there is displacement of the apex laterally and inferiorly, which can be seen and also felt as a thrust. A systolic ejection murmur generally will be heard at the second interspace to the right of the sternum, with transmission out the great vessels and, if loud enough, will be accompanied by a thrill. Should the fibrous ring be some distance below the valve, the murmur may be heard best along the mid to lower left sternal border. The aortic valves remain normal and therefore an ejection click generally is not present. The ascending aorta is protected somewhat from the force of ejection through the ring by the normal aortic valves and secondary dilatation generally does not occur. For reasons that are not clear, aortic insufficiency, as recognized by a decrescendo diastolic murmur at the third and fourth interspaces to the left of the sternum, is a very common finding.

The diagnosis of discrete subvalvular stenosis can be suspected in a patient who has physical findings rather consistent with valvular aortic stenosis but who is missing an ejection click and has aortic insufficiency. Confirmation can be obtained with cardiac catheterization and more specifically with cineangiocardiography, which would demonstrate the fixed subvalvular ring. This is not demonstrated.

SUPRAVALVULAR STENOSIS

This is an uncommon form of left ventricular outflow obstruction and is presented for completeness. When present, it is commonly seen as part of a syndrome that includes mental retardation and elfin facies. Hypercalcemia and peripheral pulmonary artery stenoses frequently are present also.

The peripheral pulses are of particular interest in that the right radial pulse may be virtually normal whereas the left radial pulse will show a delayed upstroke, a prolonged peaking and a somewhat delayed downstroke. Reasons for this difference are not clear but may relate to the preferential flow of blood through the obstruction into the right-sided vessels, with subsequent dissipation of forces by the time the left brachial artery is reached. The first sound remains normal. An ejection click is not heard. Shortly after the opening of the normal aortic valves, the area of obstruction is encountered and an ejection systolic murmur, grade II/VI or louder, harsh in quality and low in pitch, will be generated. This murmur will be transmitted along the arterial vessels but preferentially into the right-sided rather than the left-sided arteries. If the murmur is of sufficient intensity, a thrill will be palpable and may be higher in the chest than that seen in valvular stenosis. The valves being normal, closure will be secure and the diastolic murmur of aortic insufficiency will not be heard.

The diagnosis can be suspected in a patient who has physical findings reminiscent of aortic stenosis but who also has mental retardation and elfin facies. The diagnosis can be confirmed with cardiac catheterization, during which the pressures in the left ventricle and those just distal to the aortic valve would be normal and the pressure in the arch of the aorta would be diminished. Cineangiocardiography will visually demonstrate the narrowing within the aorta itself. These events are not demonstrated.

DIFFERENTIAL DIAGNOSIS

In infancy, the patient with obstruction to left ventricular outflow must be differentiated from one having a ventricular septal defect. Although the location of the murmur may be similar, if the patient has a ventricular septal defect the quality of the murmur will be more holosystolic and will be accompanied by a thrill. In addition, a systolic ejection click will be absent. If necessary, cardiac catheterization will confirm the differential diagnosis.

PEARLS

1. Aortic stenosis is more common in males than in females.

2. Although reverse splitting of the second sound can be expected in very severe aortic stenosis, it also can be seen with a left bundle-branch block.

3. The physical findings in the infant may be different from those in the child.

4. The degree of gradient across the aortic valve cannot always be suspected on the basis of the amount of left ventricular hypertrophy on the electrocardiogram.

5. The presence of a systolic ejection click strongly suggests that the obstruction is at the valve.

6. A bicuspid aortic valve is seen quite commonly in patients with coarctation of the aorta.

CHAPTER SIX

Pulmonary Stenosis and Other Lesions Obstructive to Right Ventricular Outflow

EMBRYOLOGY

BETWEEN the 6th and 9th weeks of gestation, concomitant with the development of the truncus arteriosus, the pulmonary valve develops. It is formed by enlargement of three tubercles within the lumen of the pulmonary artery (Fig. 6–1). The tubercles grow toward the midline and are thinned by resorption of tissue. There is additional hollowing out of tissue at the superior por-

Fig. 6–1. – Demonstration of formation of the pulmonary valves within the pulmonary artery. Note the progressive proliferation of the truncoconal ridges. (The aortic valves are also demonstrated coincidentally.) (Modified from Moss, A. J., and Adams, F. H. [eds.]: *Heart Disease in Infants, Children and Adolescents* [Baltimore: The Williams & Wilkins Company, 1968], p. 16.)

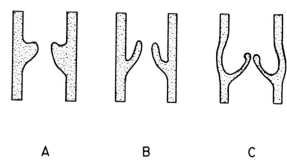

A   B   C

Fig. 6–2.—A graphic representation of the proliferation and then hollowing out of the tubercles, giving rise to the completed valve.

tion of the tubercle at its junction with the wall of the pulmonary artery, giving rise to the sinuses of the valve (Fig. 6–2).

Slightly before the development of the pulmonary valves, the infundibulum of the right ventricle is being formed from the proximal portion of the bulbus cordis.

At about the same time—the fifth to the seventh week of gestation—the aortic arch system is differentiating. The sixth arch becomes the distal portion of the pulmonary artery. Distally, it connects to the smaller pulmonary arteries, which develop from the pulmonary vascular plexus, and proximally it connects to the main pulmonary artery.

ANATOMY

Failure of normal development of the tissue-thin three leaflets of the pulmonary valve will result in an abnormality of that valve. This may present as only two leaflets that may be fused at their common commissures. Three leaflets may develop but may be thickened and partially fused at their commissures or totally fused, with no semblance of commissures, giving a cone-like, tunnel-shaped valve resembling, somewhat, the mouth of a fish. Being able to picture the narrow orifice of either two or three leaflets, which grossly restricts valve motion, will aid in the understanding of the dynamics of the lesion.

If there is insufficient resorption of tissue in the bulbus cordis, an area of infundibular hypertrophy will result. In addition, abnormal bands of muscle may be laid down within the body of the right ventricle.

Last, in the development of the peripheral pulmonary arteries, the hollowing out of those vessels may be interfered with, giving rise to multiple areas of stenosis.

HEMODYNAMICS

A common denominator in each of these lesions, regardless of its specific location, is an obstruction to right ventricular systolic ejection. This effectively presents a pressure burden—enormous at times—on the right ventricle. This is conceptualized in the following mnemonic, which demonstrates an obstruction at the pulmonary valve but is applicable in principal, regardless of the location of the obstruction.

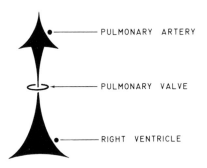

PULMONARY ARTERY

PULMONARY VALVE

RIGHT VENTRICLE

The arrow represents blood flowing from the right ventricle through the narrowed valve into the pulmonary artery. The tip of the arrow has passed the obstructed valve, dissipating its energy into the pulmonary artery. The base of the arrow represents the force required to overcome the area of obstruction.

If the blood flow is followed with the mnemonic in mind, the effect on the size of chambers and vessels of the heart can be demonstrated by the following diagram:

RIGHT ATRIUM → ↑	LEFT ATRIUM →
RIGHT VENTRICLE ↑	LEFT VENTRICLE →
MAIN PULMONARY ARTERY ↑	AORTA →
LEFT PULMONARY ARTERY ↑	
PULMONARY VESSELS →	

The arrows represent alteration in the size of a chamber or a vessel as follows:

→ Unchanged
↑ Increased

In valvular pulmonary stenosis, this effect is directly transferable to the chest x-ray. One would expect right ventricular enlargement, main pulmonary artery enlargement, normal pulmonary vascularity and a normal left side (Fig. 6–3). The electrocardiogram also would be expected to show right ventricular hypertrophy (Fig. 6–4). When severe stenosis is present, right atrial hypertrophy will be seen also.

If the obstruction is in the infundibulum, the right ventricular force will be dissipated through the elongated area of obstruc-

Fig. 6–3.—Chest roentgenograms of a patient with valvular pulmonary stenosis. Note the normal right atrium, the enlarged right ventricle impinging on the retrosternal space and the dilated pulmonary artery. The pulmonary vessels are normal. *RA* = right atrium, *RV* = right ventricle, *PA* = pulmonary artery, *PV* = pulmonary vessels.

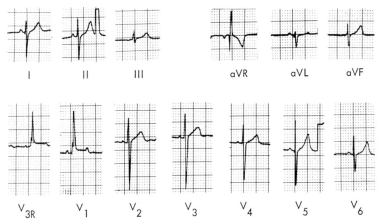

Fig. 6–4.—Electrocardiogram of a 4-year-old patient with valvular pulmonary stenosis. The salient features are the dominant S_I and R_{III} — right axis deviation. There also is a dominant R wave in V_1 and S wave in $V_{5, 6}$, which is interpretable as right ventricular hypertrophy. The T wave in V_1 is also upright.

tion in such a way as to eliminate the abnormal dilatation of the pulmonary artery distal to the valve. On x-ray, the pulmonary artery would not be dilated. The electrocardiogram would continue to show the abnormal right-sided work load. This is not demonstrated.

Obstruction within the ventricular chamber itself would reflect in the electrocardiogram and chest x-ray in a fashion similar to obstruction at the infundibulum.

Stenosis of the peripheral pulmonary arteries will have variable radiographic and electrocardiographic findings, depending on the severity and location of the lesions.

CLINICAL APPLICATION

Although the site of obstruction is not critical in understanding certain principles, it does affect the details of clinical interpretation and the precise diagnosis. Therefore, each variety of right ventricular obstruction will be discussed individually.

Valvular Stenosis

Valvular stenosis may be mild to very severe. An estimate as to the severity can be made on the basis of the physical examination. In severe stenosis, the excursion of the valve is most limited and the murmur will begin with the first heart sound, ascending in crescendo throughout most of systole, becoming decrescendo, ending at and obscuring the pulmonary component of the second sound. The murmur will be grade IV/VI or greater, generating a palpable thrill at the second left interspace. It will be transmitted along the pulmonary vessels, so it can be expected to be heard in the back. Ejection time will be delayed, resulting in a delayed closure of the pulmonary valve. The significantly restricted excursion capability of the stenosed valve will diminish the intensity of its closure. This will result in a very widely split second sound with a diminished pulmonary component. The splitting may be recognized only on a phonocardiogram. A right ventricular lift usually would be felt.

If the stenosis is moderate, the first sound will occur and the valves will open, giving rise to an ejection click, which will be followed promptly by the systolic ejection murmur. This will tend to peak somewhat earlier in systole and will decrescendo, ending after the aortic component of the second sound but before the pulmonary component. The splitting of the second sound may not be as wide and the intensity of the closure of the pulmonary valve not as diminished.

The relationship between the severity of stenosis, the ejection click and the ejection murmur now can be applied to mild pulmonary stenosis. The milder the stenosis the wider will be the interval between the first sound and the ejection click, and the peak of the ejection murmur will be reached earlier, with a decrescendo phase ending either with the aortic closure or before the aortic closure. This concept is described beautifully by Perloff and is shown in Figure 6–5.

Cardiac catheterization will be useful in confirming the clinical impression and, based on the height of the right ventricular pressure, the degree of severity (Table 6–1). Angiocardiography will show the nature of the stenotic valves.

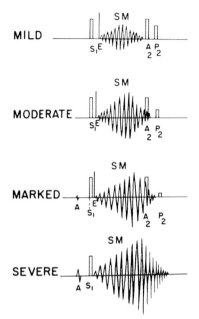

Fig. 6–5.—A graphic representation of the relationship between the first sound, the ejection click, the systolic, the aortic and pulmonic components of the second sound and the appearance of an atrial sound in pulmonary stenosis. (See text for explanation.) S_1 = first sound, E = ejection click, SM = systolic, A_2 = aortic component, P_2 = pulmonic component, A = atrial sound. (Modified from Perloff, J. K.: *The Clinical Recognition of Congenital Heart Disease* [Philadelphia: W. B. Saunders Company, 1973], p. 145.)

Malignant Pulmonary Stenosis

There occurs in the infant an unusual and particularly devastating form of severe valvular pulmonary stenosis. It is a unique expression of valvular stenosis and is best described as it presents clinically.

At about 6 months of age or so, the severe stenosis so greatly restricts right ventricular output that acute and sudden right heart failure ensues. The resulting increase in end-diastolic pressure causes tricuspid insufficiency and a concomitant increase in

TABLE 6–1.–IDEALIZED CARDIAC CATHETERIZATION DATA
IN A CHILD WITH VALVULAR PULMONARY STENOSIS*

SITE	PRESSURE (mm Hg)		OXYGEN SATURATION (%)	
	Normal	Patient	Normal	Patient
Superior vena cava			70	70
Inferior vena cava			74	74
Right atrium	a = 5 v = 3 m = 4	a = 9 v = 6 m = 6	72	72
Right ventricle	25/2	80/4	72	72
Main pulmonary artery	25/12	15/9	72	72
Left pulmonary artery	25/12	15/9	72	72
Systemic artery	120/80	120/80	97	97

*The salient features are an increase in pressure in the right ventricle and a slight decrease in pressure in the pulmonary arteries. There is no change in oxygen saturations.

right atrial pressure. Dilatation of the right atrium follows, with the foramen ovale becoming incompetent. A right-to-left shunt follows. The previously established systolic ejection murmur diminishes acutely and cyanosis occurs along with the expected clinical signs of congestive heart failure.

Usually, the diagnosis of pulmonary stenosis had been considered prior to the acute episode. If not, the diagnosis can be established with cardiac catheterization and angiocardiography. Although this is about the same time that patients with tetralogy of Fallot also become cyanotic, the appearance of congestive heart failure supports the diagnosis of pulmonary stenosis with intact septum in contradistinction to tetralogy of Fallot.

Anomalous Muscle Bundles

These muscle bundles effectively divide the right ventricle into two chambers. The inflow portion near the tricuspid valve would be the high-pressure area whereas the outflow portion below the pulmonary valve would be the low-pressure area. The valves themselves and the pulmonary artery will be normal. As the ventricle begins systole, the obstruction is encountered immediately, no ejection click is heard and the murmur will begin with the first sound and end before the second sound. Its location will be lower on the chest in the vicinity of the third or fourth interspace. The intensity of the murmur will vary with the degree of stenosis, being as small as grade II/VI or as great as grade IV/VI. A thrill will be palpable with the latter. If the obstruction is severe, the proximal portion of the right ventricle will be greatly hypertrophied and will impinge on the retrosternal space. This would cause a bulging of the lower portion of the left precordium. Its contractions would be felt as a right ventricular lift or heave.

The closure of the pulmonary valve may be delayed because of prolongation of right ventricular ejection time. The poststenotic force of blood flow is dissipated in the infundibular area of the right ventricle, which, when combined with normal valve tissue, would give rise to a normal intensity of valvular closure. One then would expect a wide splitting of the second sound, with a normal pulmonary component.

This lesion is not easily differentiated from other forms of right ventricular obstruction, and cardiac catheterization with angiocardiography is necessary to make the differentiation. Pressure tracings will show the differences within the right ventricle and an angiogram from the right atrium will visually demonstrate the area of obstruction.

Infundibular Stenosis

Obstruction in the infundibulum may be due to either a discrete fibrous ring just below the pulmonary valve or thickened, elongated muscle tissue. In the first instance, the findings will be quite similar to those of valvular pulmonary stenosis. However, since the valves themselves and the pulmonary artery itself are normal, an ejection click will not be heard and the intensity of closure of the valves will be normal. The time of closure, however, will be delayed for the same reasons as with infundibular or valvular stenosis. The physical findings of muscular infundibular stenosis will be quite similar to those of the anomalous muscle bundles just described. The murmur, however, may be slightly higher on the chest.

Once more, cardiac catheterization will be required to define the location and nature of the obstruction. Pressure curves will show an abrupt change from the low values in the pulmonary artery to the high values in the right ventricle if the obstruction is a fixed ring (quite like valvular stenosis). If there is an elongated area of hypertrophied infundibulum, the pressure curve will show an area of slightly elevated right ventricular pressure between the low pulmonary artery values and the markedly higher values in the body of the right ventricle near the tricuspid valve.

Peripheral Pulmonary Artery Stenosis

As implied in this heading, the pulmonary arteries themselves can be stenosed. As demonstrated in Figure 6–6, these areas of stenoses may be single or multiple, localized or diffuse. In all instances, the murmur is a result of turbulence through the obstruction. The point of maximal intensity of the murmur will depend on the location of the obstruction, and the transmission of the murmur will be distal to the obstruction throughout the pulmonary arterial tree. The murmur of the usual multiple peripheral pulmonary artery stenosis is heard at the second interspace, to the left and right of the sternum, and is transmitted well beneath each clavicle, into each axilla and throughout the back. The murmur generally is systolic in time and ejection in character. It is possible, however, for turbulence to occur in both systole and diastole, and a murmur reminiscent of a ductus can be heard.

Because the pulmonary valves are normal and the obstruction is distal to them, no ejection click is heard. Since the obstruction will result in a high-pressure area proximal to it but distal to the pulmonary valves, it can be anticipated that normal closure of the valves will occur, but the intensity of the pulmonary component may be increased, depending on the severity of the stenosis.

Although the electrocardiogram may show right ventricular hypertrophy, its relationship to the degree of severity is not clearly as accurate as with valvular stenosis. A chest x-ray will not be particularly useful in identifying this entity. Cardiac catheterization and angiocardiography, however, will be useful in defining the specific location and nature of the lesions.

TYPE I

SINGLE, CENTRAL STENOSIS

A

B

TYPE II

BIFURCATION STENOSIS

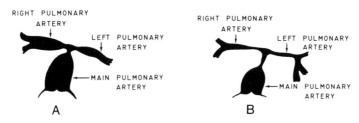

A

B

TYPE III

MULTIPLE, PERIPHERAL STENOSIS

TYPE IV

CENTRAL+PERIPHERAL STENOSIS

Fig. 6—6. — Classification of peripheral pulmonary artery stenosis. (Modified from Gay, Franch, Shuford and Rogers: Am J. Roentgenol. 90:599, 1963.)

A patient can be suspected of having an obstruction to right ventricular outflow if he is asymptomatic, has prominent left chest with a palpable heave, a systolic ejection click at the second interspace to the left of the sternum, a widely duplicated second sound with a diminished pulmonary component, a systolic ejection murmur loudest at the second and third interspaces to the left of the sternum that transmits to the back and a thrill at the site of the murmur. The chest x-ray will show right ventricular enlargement, a dilated main pulmonary artery and normal vascular markings. The electrocardiogram will show right ventricular hypertrophy. The precise site of obstruction can be determined with cardiac catheterization, during which an elevated pressure will be found proximal to and a diminished pressure distal to the site of obstruction. Cineangiocardiography will clarify the nature of the obstruction.

DIFFERENTIAL DIAGNOSIS

The patient with obstruction to right ventricular outflow must be differentiated from a patient with an atrial septal defect, a patent ductus arteriosus and an innocent murmur.

The patient with an atrial septal defect will have a murmur ejection in quality and systolic in time at the same location but it will be softer in intensity and will have a widely split second sound that does not vary with respiration.

The patient with a patent ductus arteriosus can be confused with one having pulmonary stenosis only if the diastolic portion of the murmur is not present consistently. If that is the case, cardiac catheterization may be necessary to effect the differential.

The patient with an innocent murmur has a softer murmur, a perfectly normal second sound, a normal chest x-ray and a normal electrocardiogram.

PEARLS

1. Valvular pulmonary stenosis is more common in males than in females.

2. Pulmonary artery stenosis is seen frequently with rubella syndrome. These patients will not be well developed and well nourished.

3. Mild valvular pulmonary stenosis may be difficult to distinguish from an innocent murmur.

4. There is good correlation between the degree of stenosis and the degree of right ventricular hypertrophy on the electrocardiogram.

CHAPTER SEVEN

Coarctation of the Aorta

EMBRYOLOGY

BETWEEN the fifth and seventh weeks of gestation, the aortic arch develops. This begins as six paired arches proliferating from the distal end of the truncus arteriosus. While the right fourth arch participates in the development of the right subclavian artery, the left fourth arch becomes the definitive aortic arch connecting with the left dorsal aorta to complete the entire aorta (Fig. 7 – 1).

ANATOMY

For reasons that are not known, the area of the aorta near the insertion of the ductus arteriosus may develop improperly, leav-

Fig. 7–1. – Diagrammatic representation of the formation of the aortic arch. Panel **A** shows the primitive six arches originating from the distal end of the truncus arteriosus. Panel **B** shows the definitive form of the aorta, indicating its origin in the fourth arch.

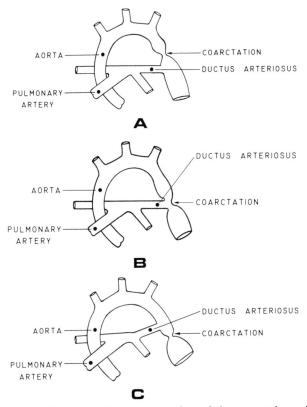

Fig. 7–2. – Diagrammatic representation of the anatomic variations of coarctation of the aorta as it relates to the location of the ductus arteriosus. **A,** preductal. **B,** at the ductus. **C,** postductal.

ing a restricted lumen. This can take place proximal to, at or distal to the insertion of the ductus arteriosus (Fig. 7–2). It is on this basis that a classification of preductal or postductal coarctation of the aorta has been established. The entire aorta from the aortic valve into the abdominal aorta can be affected, but only the most common site in the vicinity of the ductus will be considered. The precise location of the coarctation will affect the entire clinical picture; therefore, each will be discussed individually.

PREDUCTAL COARCTATION OF THE AORTA

Hemodynamics

The coarctation obstructs flow from the proximal portion of the aorta to its distal portion. If the coarctation is proximal to the insertion of the ductus arteriosus, the lower half of the body will be supplied by the right ventricle through the ductus. The upper half of the body will be supplied by the left ventricle, and collateral circulation will not be stimulated during fetal life. After birth, the circuitry persists and can be conceptualized in the mnemonic

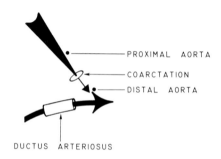

The arrows represent blood entering the descending aorta from the right ventricle through the ductus (heavy arrow) and to a much lesser degree from the ascending aorta (thin arrow). If the flow is followed with the relative size of the arrows kept in mind, the effect on the heart can be demonstrated by the following diagram:

RIGHT ATRIUM →	LEFT ATRIUM → ↑
RIGHT VENTRICLE ↑	LEFT VENTRICLE → ↑
MAIN PULMONARY ARTERY ↑	ASCENDING AORTA →
PULMONARY VESSELS →	DESCENDING AORTA ↑

The arrows represent alteration in the size of a vessel or a chamber as follows:

→ Unchanged
↑ Increased

Translated to the chest x-ray, one might expect a normal right atrium, enlarged right ventricle, a full pulmonary artery segment

Fig. 7–3.—Chest roentgenograms of a newborn with preductal coarctation of the aorta. Although the right atrium and the right ventricle are labeled, it would be more accurate to state that generalized cardiomegaly is present with normal pulmonary vascularity. *RA* = right atrium, *RV* = right ventricle.

and a prominent descending aorta. The left atrium and the left ventricle usually are unimpressive in size. The arch of the aorta might be diminished in size but this usually is not apparent on the x-ray. Parenthetically, since this variation almost always presents in the newborn period and since specific chamber enlargement is quite difficult to recognize in this age range, the usual chest x-ray may show only cardiomegaly (Fig. 7–3). The electrocardiogram will consistently show right ventricular hypertrophy (Fig. 7–4).

Clinical Application

The patient—usually an infant—with preductal coarctation of the aorta should have differential cyanosis. The lower half of the body is being supplied by the right ventricle and should be cyanotic whereas the upper half of the body is being supplied by the left ventricle and should be totally oxygenated. Theoretically, this is the case and chemically can be shown to exist but visually occurs only rarely. (This is a common examination question.) Hypertension in the upper extremities and a lower pressure in the lower extremities can be expected. Because the right ventricle has been perfusing the lower half of the body throughout fe-

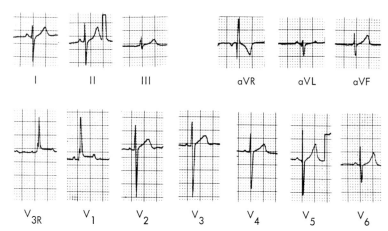

Fig. 7–4. — Electrocardiogram of an infant with preductal coarctation of the aorta. The salient features are the dominant S_1 and R_{III} — right axis deviation. There also is a dominant R wave in V_1 and S wave in $V_{5,\,6}$, which is interpretable as right ventricular hypertrophy. The T wave in V_1 is also upright.

TABLE 7–1.—IDEALIZED CARDIAC CATHETERIZATION DATA IN AN INFANT WITH PREDUCTAL COARCTATION OF THE AORTA*

SITE	PRESSURE (mm Hg)		OXYGEN SATURATION (%)	
	Normal	Patient	Normal	Patient
Superior vena cava			70	70
Inferior vena cava			74	74
Right atrium	a=5 v=3 m=4		72	72
Right ventricle	25/2	90/2	72	72
Main pulmonary artery	25/2	90/50	72	72
Left atrium	a=5 v=7 m=6	a=5 v=7 m=6	97	97
Left ventricle	90/5	120/5	97	97
Ascending aorta	90/50	120/50	97	97
Descending aorta	90/50	65/50	97	80

*The salient features are elevated pressures in the right ventricle and the main pulmonary artery. The pressure in the left ventricle and the ascending aorta is even higher. The pressure in the descending aorta is diminished. The oxygen saturation in the descending aorta is diminished.

tal life and continues to do so after birth, the femoral pulses will be present but diminished in amplitude, but their onset will be delayed when compared to the radial pulse. Normally, no murmur is present. This is because collateral vessels normally are not present in any significant degree and there is very little antegrade flow through the coarcted segment. A bicuspid aortic valve is a frequent coexisting lesion. If stenotic, its presence may be recognized by an ejection systolic murmur heard at the fourth interspace to the left of the sternum, with some transmission to the second interspace to the right of the sternum. The second sound will be closely split, with an intensification of the pulmonary component. This event is related to the persistence of fetal pulmonary hypertension.

Fig. 7–5. — An enlargement of a single frame of a 35-mm cineangiocardiogram performed in a newborn with preductal coarctation of the aorta. Note the insertion of the ductus arteriosus into the descending aorta distal to the site of the coarctation. *DA* = ductus arteriosus, *CA* = coarctation of the aorta, *DAo* = descending aorta, *RPA* = right pulmonary artery, *LPA* = left pulmonary artery.

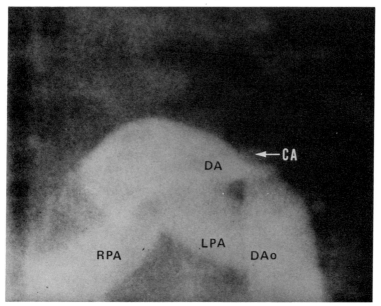

If the patient is in congestive heart failure with poor cardiac output, the classic relationship of pulses and blood pressure in the upper and lower extremities will be obscured. Therefore, it makes re-examination of the patient, when compensated, an absolute necessity.

Therefore, an infant can be suspected of having preductal coarctation of the aorta if he gets into early difficulty with congestive heart failure, demonstrates cyanosis of the lower half of the body, has prominent radial pulses with hypertension in the upper extremities and diminished femoral pulses and blood pressure in the lower extremities, right ventricular hypertrophy in the electrocardiogram and cardiomegaly in the chest x-ray. If in doubt, the diagnosis can be proved with cardiac catheterization, during which the desaturation in the descending aorta and the relative hypertension in the ascending aorta will be shown (Table 7 – 1). Angiocardiography will clarify the pathology (Fig. 7 – 5).

POSTDUCTAL COARCTATION OF THE AORTA

Hemodynamics

The coarctation obstructs flow from the proximal portion of the aorta to its distal portion. With the coarctation being distal to the insertion of the ductus arteriosus, right ventricular flow will have been into the ascending aorta throughout all of fetal life. The presence of the coarctation would require the development of collateral circulation during fetal life to permit perfusion of the lower half of the body. This is indeed the case, and is demonstrated in the mnemonic

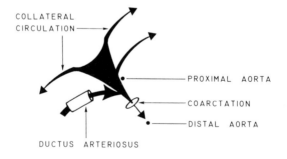

COLLATERAL CIRCULATION

PROXIMAL AORTA

COARCTATION

DISTAL AORTA

DUCTUS ARTERIOSUS

The heavy arrow represents blood flowing through the ductus into the proximal aorta. The coarctation restricts antegrade flow, as shown by the thin arrow in the distal aorta, and stimulates proximal flow, as shown by the multiple arrows in the collateral circulation. In the older infant or young child, the ductus normally closes and the infantile pulmonary hypertension resolves. If these facts are remembered and if the flow of blood now is followed with the mnemonic in mind, the effect on the heart and vessels can be demonstrated by the following diagram:

RIGHT ATRIUM →	LEFT ATRIUM → ↑
RIGHT VENTRICLE →	LEFT VENTRICLE ↑
MAIN PULMONARY ARTERY →	ASCENDING AORTA → ↑
PULMONARY VESSELS →	DESCENDING AORTA ↑

The arrows represent alteration in the size of a chamber or a vessel as follows:

→ Unchanged
↑ Increased

Translated to the chest x-ray, one would expect the right side of the heart to be normal, some possible enlargement of the left

Fig. 7–6. — Chest roentgenogram of a child with a postductal coarctation of the aorta. Note the indentation of the aorta resembling a figure 3. This is demonstrated in line form in the right-hand panel. *AAo* = ascending aorta, *CA* = coarctation of the aorta, *DAo* = descending aorta.

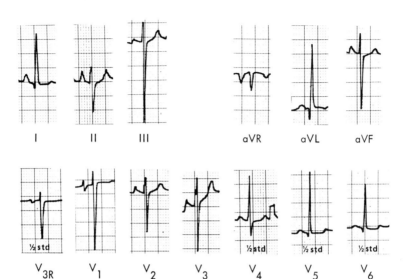

Fig. 7–7.—Electrocardiogram of a child with postductal coarctation of the aorta. The salient features are a dominant R_I and S_{III}—left axis deviation. There also is a deep S wave in lead V_1 and a very tall R wave in leads $V_{5, 6}$, which is interpretable as left ventricular hypertrophy.

atrium, an enlarged left ventricle and a dilated ascending aorta. The descending aorta would also show poststenotic dilatation and, on occasion, that relationship will be visible on the chest x-ray, resembling a figure 3. (Fig. 7–6). The electrocardiogram would demonstrate varying degrees of left ventricular hypertrophy (Fig. 7–7).

Clinical Application

These patients are uniformly pink. Pulses in the upper extremities are full whereas those in the lower extremities are diminished to absent. The blood pressure in the arms is elevated whereas that in the legs is diminished. If the orifice of the coarctation is sufficient to permit flow through it, an ejection murmur occurring after the first sound and in the middle of systole may well be heard along the upper left paravertebral area. A bruit will be heard representing collateral flow through the dilated intercostal arteries throughout the entire posterior chest and through the dilated internal mammary arteries throughout the anterior chest. If a bicuspid aortic valve is coexistent and stenotic, a harsh grade I-II/VI ejection systolic murmur will be heard at the second interspace to the right of the sternum, transmitting into the neck vessels. This murmur may be preceded by a systolic ejection click heard at the fourth interspace to the left of the sternum. It should be remembered that the click is heard over the site of the aortic valve itself and that the murmur is a transmitted sound of turbulent blood flow in the ascending aorta after it has passed the stenotic valve. Should the bicuspid valve be insufficient, a high-pitched decrescendo early to mid-diastolic murmur will be heard at the left third and fourth interspaces. The second sound generally is normal, with variable splitting and normal components. If the pressure in the ascending aorta is very high, the aortic component of the second sound should be increased in absolute intensity.

The infant with a postductal coarctation of the aorta follows one of two courses. Within the first 3 months of life, he may have congestive heart failure, presenting with the usual symp-

TABLE 7–2.—IDEALIZED CARDIAC CATHETERIZATION DATA IN A CHILD WITH POSTDUCTAL COARCTATION OF THE AORTA*

SITE	PRESSURE (mm Hg)		OXYGEN SATURATION (%)	
	Normal	Patient	Normal	Patient
Superior vena cava			70	70
Inferior vena cava			74	74
Right atrium	a = 5 v = 3 m = 4	a = 5 v = 3 m = 4	72	72
Right ventricle	25/2	25/2	72	72
Main pulmonary artery	25/12	25/12	72	72
Left atrium	a = 5 v = 7 m = 6	a = 5 v = 7 m = 6	97	97
Left ventricle	110/5	160/5	97	97
Ascending aorta	110/70	160/70	97	97
Descending aorta	110/70	70/50	97	97

*The salient feature is the presence of elevated pressures in the left ventricle and the ascending aorta with diminished pressures in the descending aorta. The oxygen saturations are entirely normal.

toms of cough and signs of tachypnea, dyspnea, tachycardia and hepatosplenomegaly. At this time, the classic findings of full pulses and hypertension in the upper extremities and diminished pulses and blood pressure in the lower extremities may be obscured because of poor cardiac output. After the compensation, the classic findings will be more apparent and therefore re-examination is mandatory. Cardiac catheterization usually is not necessary unless there is strong suspicion of significant coexisting lesions. If done, the difference in pressures in the ascending and descending aorta will be demonstrated (Table 7 – 2). Angiocardiography will demonstrate the pathology (Fig. 7 – 8). The majority of patients, however, accommodate to the coarctation and grow without trouble. The diagnosis can be established on

Fig. 7–8. – Enlargement of a single frame of a 35-mm cineangiocardiogram performed in a child with postductal coarctation of the aorta. Note the site of the coarctation. No ductus is seen because it has closed spontaneously. *AAo* = ascending aorta, *CA* = coarctation of the aorta, *DAo* = descending aorta.

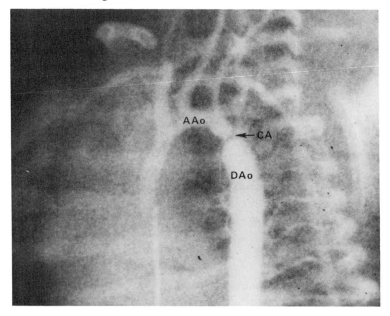

the basis of the physical examination, with lesser support from the chest x-ray and the electrocardiogram. The exact site of the coarctation in the thoracic aorta can, in fact, be suspected on the basis of palpation alone. If a pulse is palpable in the right arm and absent in the left arm and legs, the coarctation is either proximal to or at the site of the left subclavian artery. If a pulse is palpable in the left arm and absent in the right arm and legs, the coarctation is distal to the left subclavian artery, but there is an anomalous right subclavian artery originating distal to the site of the coarctation. The presence of pulses in the right arm and right carotid but the absence of pulses in the left carotid, left arm and legs suggests that the coarctation is at the isthmus.

DIFFERENTIAL DIAGNOSIS

The lesion is not confused with many others. It must be differentiated from other noncardiac causes of hypertension, such as essential hypertension, renal pathology and pheochromocytoma.

PEARLS

1. Coarctation of the aorta is more common in males than in females.

2. Coarctation can occur at any site in the aorta, and abdominal location should be looked for routinely.

3. Rib notching, a common finding in the older patient with coarctation of the aorta, normally does not occur before 8 years of age. It is a function of physical erosion of the undersurface of the ribs due to intercostal collateral circulation.

4. Bicuspid aortic valve occurs in approximately 50% of patients as a coexisting lesion.

5. Coarctation of the aorta is the most common cardiac abnormality in patients with Turner's syndrome.

CHAPTER EIGHT

Tetralogy of Fallot

EMBRYOLOGY

TOWARD the end of the third week and into the fourth, the common trunk normally is divided into the pulmonary artery and the aorta. This is accomplished by the development of the truncoconal ridges, which grow caudad in a spiral fashion, resulting in the posterior lateral origin of the aorta and the anterior medial origin of the pulmonary artery (Fig. 8–1). This septum fuses with the bulbar ridges, which, in turn, participate with the endocardial cushions and membranous proliferation from the ventricular septum to form the definitive closure of the interventricular septum (Fig. 8–2).

Fig. 8–1. – Diagrammatic representation of the division of the truncus arteriosus (**A**) into the aorta and pulmonary artery (**C**). Panel **B** shows the septation and the spiral direction of the pulmonary artery and the aorta. *PA* = pulmonary artery, *Ao* = aorta.

Fig. 8–2. – Schematic representation of the role of the bulbus cordis in the formation of the interventricular septum. (See text for explanation.)

Between the fourth and eighth weeks of gestation, the single ventricular chamber is effectively divided into two. This is accomplished by fusion of the membranous portion of the ventricular septum, the endocardial cushions and the bulbus cordis (the proximal portion of the truncus arteriosus). The muscular portion of the ventricular septum grows cephalad as each ventricular chamber enlarges, eventually meeting with the right and left

Fig. 8–3. – Schematic representation of the formation of the interventricular septum. **A,** 30 days; **B,** 33 days; **C,** 37 days; **D,** newborn. (See text for explanation.) (Modified from Moss, A. J., and Adams, F. H. [eds.]: *Heart Disease in Infants, Children and Adolescents* [Baltimore: The Williams & Wilkins Company, 1968], p. 16.)

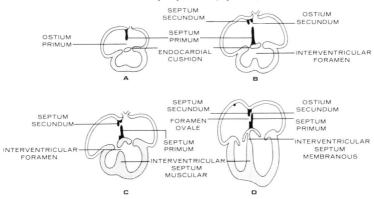

ridges of the bulbus cordis. The right ridge fuses with the tricuspid valve and the endocardial cushion, thus separating the pulmonary valve from the tricuspid valve. The left ridge fuses with a ridge of the interventricular septum, leaving the aortic ring in continuity with the mitral ring. The endocardial cushions are concomitantly developing and ultimately fuse with the bulbar ridges and the muscular portion of the septum. The final closure and separation of the two ventricles is made by the fibrous tissue of the membranous portion of the interventricular septum (Fig. 8 – 3).

ANATOMY

There are essentially two theories that are proposed in an attempt to explain the tetralogy of Fallot. The first relates merely to an abnormality in the septation of the truncus. It is postulated that if this septation is asymmetric, the two great vessels will be of unequal size. Because of the asymmetry, that portion of the septum that participates in closure of the atrioventricular area will not be available and a ventricular septal defect will result. The asymmetry will also lead to a greater than normal amount of tissue in the infundibulum of the right ventricle, which then would account for the infundibular stenosis. The other theory relates the entire clinical picture to an abnormality in development of the infundibular area of the right ventricle. It is believed that the infundibular stenosis restricts blood flow through the pulmonary artery during fetal life, causing it to be smaller than normal at the time of birth. Increased blood flow through the aorta during fetal life causes it to be large at the time of birth. The improper development of the infundibular area also disturbs the normal completion of the atrioventricular canal and a resultant ventricular septal defect occurs.

Whichever theory is accepted, there results a consistent hypertrophy of the crista supraventricularis, a frequent hypoplasia of the pulmonary valve annulus with stenosis of the pulmonary valves themselves and a ventricular septal defect located below the crista supraventricularis generally approximating the size of the aorta. The crista supraventricularis, by definition, is a muscular ridge located below the pulmonary valves separating the infundibulum from the remainder of the right ventricular cavity (Fig. 8–4).

Traditionally, tetralogy of Fallot has been defined as consisting of four basic anatomic abnormalities: infundibular stenosis, ventricular septal defect, right ventricular hypertrophy and overriding or dextroposition of the aorta. From an anatomic standpoint, this remains the case, but from a physiologic standpoint it is my belief that only the infundibular stenosis and the ventricular septal defect are of importance. The right ventricular hypertrophy is secondary to the obstruction to right ventricular ejection and the aorta receives poorly oxygenated blood because

Fig. 8–4. – Diagrammatic representation of the appearance of the crista supraventricularis and its parietal and septal bands in a normal patient and in a patient with tetralogy of Fallot. **A,** normal – lateral view; **B,** normal – AP view; **C,** tetralogy of Fallot – lateral view; **D,** tetralogy of Fallot – AP view. Note the increased size in the parietal band and septal band and the presence of a ventricular septal defect in **C** and **D.** *PB* = parietal band, *SB* = septal band, *RV* = right ventricle, *I* = infundibulum.

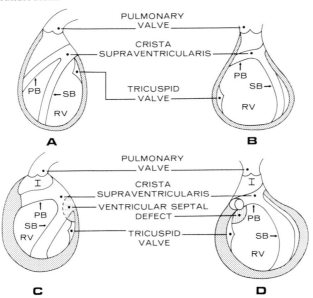

of the obstruction of right ventricular ejection in the presence of a ventricular septal defect without regard to the degree of physical overriding of the aorta.

If the physiologic parameters are accepted for the criteria of diagnosis, one patient may have very mild infundibular stenosis, be minimally cyanotic and be considered as having a "pink tetralogy" whereas another would have obliteration of the outflow tract, be exceptionally cyanotic and be considered as having pulmonary atresia. In fact, such a panorama exists. It has been my choice, however, to use the remainder of the chapter to deal with what might loosely be called "classic tetralogy of Fallot," in which infundibular stenosis, a ventricular septal defect approximating the size of the aorta and right ventricular pressures that are systemic in height are present. Hypoplasia of the pulmonary valve annulus and stenosis of the valves are present so commonly as to be considered virtually an intregal part of the pathologic complex.

HEMODYNAMICS

The patient with tetralogy of Fallot has diminished blood flow to the lungs and increased blood flow to the body. This is demonstrated in the mnemonic

The small arrow entering the pulmonary artery represents diminished blood flow through the stenotic infundibulum. The heavier arrow represents flow of venous blood through the ven-

tricular septal defect into the aorta. The thick black area identified as the right ventricle indicates the increased pressure in that
chamber. If the blood flow is followed with mnemonic in mind,
the effect on the heart can be demonstrated by the following diagram:

RIGHT ATRIUM → ↑	LEFT ATRIUM →
RIGHT VENTRICLE ↑	LEFT VENTRICLE →
MAIN PULMONARY ARTERY ↓	AORTA ↑
PULMONARY VESSELS ↓	

The arrows represent alteration in the size of a chamber or
a vessel as follows:

→ Unchanged
↑ Increased
↓ Decreased

This information can be translated to the chest x-ray, where
one would expect to see possible enlargement of the right
atrium, definite enlargement of the right ventricle, a small main
pulmonary artery and a normal left atrium and left ventricle —

Fig. 8–5. — Chest roentgenograms of a patient with tetralogy of Fallot.
Note the enlarged right atrium and right ventricle and decreased pul-
monary vessels. The over-all appearance is that of a boot-shaped heart.
RA = right atrium, *RV* = right ventricle, *PV* = pulmonary vessels.

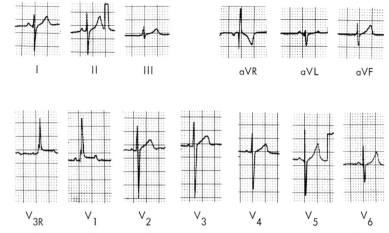

| I | II | III | aVR | aVL | aVF |

| V_{3R} | V_1 | V_2 | V_3 | V_4 | V_5 | V_6 |

Fig. 8–6. — Electrocardiogram of a patient with tetralogy of Fallot. The salient features are the dominant S_I and R_{III} — right axis deviation. There also is a dominant R wave in V_1 and S wave in $V_{5, 6}$, which is interpretable as right ventricular hypertrophy. The T wave in V_1 is also upright.

recognized as a boot-shaped heart. The aorta would be enlarged. In 25% of patients, the aorta arches to the right (Fig. 8–5). The electrocardiogram would show right ventricular hypertrophy (Fig. 8–6).

CLINICAL APPLICATION

It is believed by many that the infundibular hypertrophy intrinsic to tetralogy of Fallot increases progressively with age and, as such, increases the right-to-left shunting through the ventricular septal defect. If this is the case, it can offer an explanation for the delayed appearance of cyanosis. With time and persistent cyanosis, the fingers and toes become clubbed and squatting occurs. As the right ventricle hypertrophies, it encroaches on the retrosternal space, and its contractions can be felt as a heave along the left sternal border. The first sound will be normal. Generally, no ejection click will be heard. The aorta, because of its malposition, is closer to the chest wall than usual and its valve closure is heard more easily. The infundibular stenosis is responsible for a prolonged ejection time of the right ventricle, which greatly delays the closing of the pulmonary valve. The valve itself frequently is thickened and relatively immobile, causing it to close with decreased intensity. This all results in a single second sound to auscultation, which can be recorded on a phonocardiogram as a very widely duplicated event with marked diminution of the pulmonary component. The murmur, related to flow through the infundibulum, will be heard in the second and third interspaces to the left of the sternum, be systolic in time, ejection in quality and transmitted into the pulmonary vessels.

As a result of the restricted blood flow, collateral circulation through bronchial vessels or other aortic pulmonary communications develops occasionally. Its presence will be recognized as continuous murmurs, generally heard over the back.

The cyanosis is responsible for a number of secondary events. The relative hypoxemia tends to stimulate red cell production. If oral intake of iron is insufficient for the increased number of red

TABLE 8-1. – IDEALIZED CARDIAC CATHETERIZATION DATA
IN A PATIENT WITH TETRALOGY OF FALLOT*

SITE	PRESSURE (mm Hg)		OXYGEN SATURATION (%)	
	Normal	Patient	Normal	Patient
Superior vena cava			70	54
Inferior vena cava			74	6ſ
Right atrium	a = 5 v = 3 m = 4	a = 9 v = 7 m = 6	72	56
Right ventricle – body	25/2	120/2	72	56
Right ventricle – infundibulum	25/2	70/2	72	56
Main pulmonary artery	25/2	20/10	72	56
Systemic artery	120/80	120/80	97	80

*The salient feature is generalized low oxygen saturations on the right side of the heart with desaturation in the systemic artery. There is systemic pressure in the body of the right ventricle, diminished pressure in the infundibulum and very low pressure in the main pulmonary artery. There also is a slight elevation of the pressure in the right atrium.

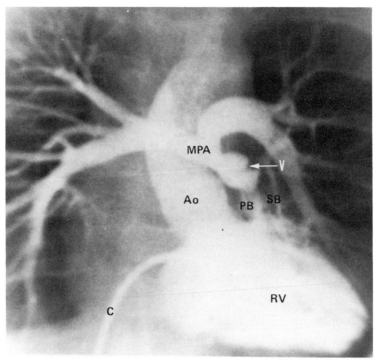

Fig. 8–7. — Enlargement of a single frame from a cineangiocardiogram, in the AP projection, in a patient with tetralogy of Fallot. Note the narrow infundibulum bordered by the parietal band and septal band, the small pulmonary valve and main pulmonary artery and the enlarged aorta, which is being filled from the right ventricle. C = catheter, RV = right ventricle, PB = parietal band, SB = septal band, V = pulmonary valve, MPA = main pulmonary artery, Ao = aorta.

cells, an iron-deficiency anemia will result. This diagnosis may be elusive because the patient may have a normal hemoglobin for his age but still have a relative anemia. Therefore, a hematocrit and red cell indices must also be obtained to ensure an accurate hematologic evaluation. The polycythemia so commonly present increases the risk of developing a cerebral thrombosis and hemiplegia. Transient cerebral ischemia can occur, leading to paleness, limpness and unconsciousness—the spells of tetralogy of Fallot. The right-to-left shunting through the

A   **B**

Fig. 8–8.—Enlargement of two frames from a cineangiocardiogram, in the lateral projection, in a patient with tetralogy of Fallot. In panel **A,** note the presence of the small main pulmonary artery arising from the right ventricle with the presence of the thickened crista supraventricularis. The ventricular septal defect is seen. In panel **B,** taken several milliseconds later, note the presence of the aorta as it fills from the right ventricle. C = catheter, RV = right ventricle, VSD = ventricular septal defect, CS = crista supraventricularis, MPA = main pulmonary artery, Ao = aorta.

ventricular septal defect increases the risk for cerebral abscesses.

The diagnosis of tetralogy of Fallot can be suspected in a patient who develops cyanosis in the middle of his first year of life, has a prominent left chest with a right ventricular heave, a single second sound, a systolic ejection murmur at the second and third interspaces to the left of the sternum, a chest x-ray showing the classic boot-shaped heart with diminished pulmonary vascular markings and an electrocardiogram with right ventricular hypertrophy. The diagnosis can be confirmed with cardiac catheterization, which will show systemic pressure in the right ventricle, diminished pressure in the infundibular area, markedly diminished pressure in the pulmonary artery and arterial desaturation (Table 8–1). Cineangiocardiography would demonstrate the ventricular septal defect, the infundibular stenosis, the small pulmonary artery and the displaced and enlarged aorta (Figs. 8–7 and 8–8).

DIFFERENTIAL DIAGNOSIS

The patient with tetralogy of Fallot must be differentiated from one having severe valvular pulmonary stenosis with an intact ventricular septum, truncus arteriosus with diminished pulmonary flow (type IV), Eisenmenger's complex, origin of both great vessels from the right ventricle with pulmonary stenosis, transposition of the great arteries with subpulmonic stenosis and ventricular septal defect and tricuspid atresia.

The patient with severe pulmonary stenosis — also called malignant pulmonary stenosis — is discussed in Chapter 6. Although he will have cyanosis at about the same age, he will be severely ill with intense congestive heart failure and diminishing murmurs. Cardiac catheterization may be necessary to define the presence of an intact ventricular septum.

On clinical grounds alone, the patient with truncus arteriosus may be quite difficult to distinguish from one having tetralogy of Fallot. Cardiac catheterization normally will permit that differentiation.

The patient with Eisenmenger's complex may be momentarily confused with one having tetralogy of Fallot. The presence of cardiomegaly and increased vascular markings in the hilar area of the lungs, as seen on chest x-ray, will be useful in the differential. Cardiac catheterization can finally delineate the two.

The patient with both great vessels arising from the right ventricle with pulmonary stenosis physiologically behaves quite like one with tetralogy of Fallot. However, basic to the lesion is separation of the normal continuity between the aortic ring and the mitral ring. This can be demonstrated on an echocardiogram or with a cineangiocardiogram.

The patient with transposition of the great arteries with ventricular septal defect and subpulmonic stenosis is discussed in detail in Chapter 10. He may be difficult to distinguish from one having tetralogy of Fallot, for both have an enlarged right ventricle, diminished pulmonary vascular markings and a single second sound. The chest x-ray and the electrocardiogram are reminiscent of each other. However, cardiac catheterization will clearly delineate the two.

The patient with tricuspid atresia will be of concern only on the basis of cyanosis, but will be easily differentiated once an electrocardiogram is done. The presence of left ventricle hypertrophy will make the distinction.

PEARLS

1. This lesion occurs equally in males and females.

2. Congestive heart failure is extraordinarily rare and its presence should direct your attention initially elsewhere.

3. An apparently normal hemoglobin in a cyanotic patient should be evaluated further for iron-deficiency anemia.

4. The appearance of cyanosis is indication enough for performing an elective cardiac catheterization.

5. A right aortic arch is seen in approximately 25% of the patients.

6. Rarely, the left pulmonary artery may be totally absent.

CHAPTER NINE

Tricuspid Atresia

EMBRYOLOGY

AT ABOUT the fifth week of gestation there is a blending of the anterior endocardial cushion, the posterior endocardial cushion, a portion of the interventricular septum and the ventricular muscle itself to form the right atrioventricular valve, also known as the tricuspid valve (Figs. 9–1 and 9–2).

The papillary muscles and the chordae tendineae arise from careful sculpturing of ventricular muscle (Fig. 9–3).

ANATOMY

If there is a disruption between the balance of proliferation and resorption of tissue, the valve leaflets will not form normally. By definition, in tricuspid atresia no vestige of valvular tissue can be found and no communication between the right atrium and the right ventricle is possible. As in almost all types of con-

Fig. 9–1.—Schematic representation of the common atrioventricular canal developing into a right and left canal. **A,** 30 days; **B,** 33 days; **C,** 35 days. (See text for explanation.) (Modified from Moss, A. J., and Adams, F. H. [eds.]: *Heart Disease in Infants, Children and Adolescents* [Baltimore: The Williams & Wilkins Company, 1968], p. 17.)

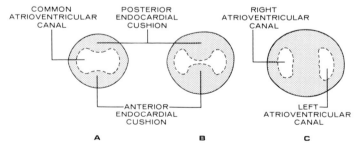

COMMON ATRIOVENTRICULAR CANAL

POSTERIOR ENDOCARDIAL CUSHION

RIGHT ATRIOVENTRICULAR CANAL

ANTERIOR ENDOCARDIAL CUSHION

LEFT ATRIOVENTRICULAR CANAL

A   B   C

Fig. 9–2.—Schematic representation of the formation of the tricuspid valve. (See text for explanation.) Identification of left-sided structures has been omitted intentionally. **A,** 37 days; **B,** newborn. (Modified from Moss, A. J., and Adams, F. H. [eds.]: *Heart Disease in Infants, Children and Adolescents* [Baltimore: The Williams & Wilkins Company, 1968], p. 16.)

genital heart disease, subclassifications exist. In tricuspid atresia, this classification depends on the relationship of the great vessels and the nature of the ventricular septum and pulmonary valve. A composite classification (Fig. 9–4) from multiple sources is as follows:

I—*Normally related great vessels*

    A. No ventricular septal defect and pulmonary atresia.

    B. Small ventricular septal defect and pulmonary stenosis.

    C. Large ventricular septal defect without pulmonary stenosis (not demonstrated).

Fig. 9–3.—Schematic representation of the formation of the atrioventricular valves and their chordae tendineae and papillary muscles. (See text for explanation.) **A** and **B,** progressive stages of development. (Modified from Moss, A. J., and Adams, F. H. [eds.]: *Heart Disease in Infants, Children and Adolescents* [Baltimore: The Williams & Wilkins Company, 1968], p. 19.)

TRICUSPID ATRESIA WITHOUT TRANSPOSITION

TRICUSPID ATRESIA WITH TRANSPOSITION

Fig. 9–4. — Classification of tricuspid atresia. **Ia,** note the absence of a ventricular septal defect and the presence of pulmonary atresia. There is a rudimentary right ventricle. **Ib,** note the presence of a small ventricular septal defect and pulmonary stenosis. The right ventricle is small. In all: *RA* = right atrium, *LA* = left atrium, *LV* = left ventricle, *AO* = aorta, *PA* = pulmonary artery. **IIa,** note the presence of a large ventricular septal defect and pulmonary atresia. The right ventricle is fairly large.

II — *Transposition of the great arteries*
   A. Ventricular septal defect and pulmonary atresia.
   B. Ventricular septal defect and pulmonary stenosis.
   C. Ventricular septal defect without pulmonary stenosis (not demonstrated).

HEMODYNAMICS

Regardless of the intricacies implicit in the classification, the flow through the heart is essentially the same and is depicted in the mnemonic

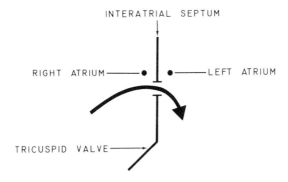

The arrow represents blood flowing from the right atrium through the interatrial septum and into the left atrium. If the blood flow is followed with this mnemonic in mind, the effect on the heart can be demonstrated by the following diagram:

RIGHT ATRIUM ↑	LEFT ATRIUM ↑
RIGHT VENTRICLE ↓	LEFT VENTRICLE ↑
PULMONARY ARTERY ↓	AORTA ↑
LUNGS ↓	

Fig. 9−5.−Chest roentgenograms of a patient with tricuspid atresia. Note the cardiomegaly, elevated apex − but due to left ventricular enlargement − and the prominent right atrium. The pulmonary markings are diminished. *LV* = left ventricle, *RA* = right atrium, *PV* = pulmonary vessels.

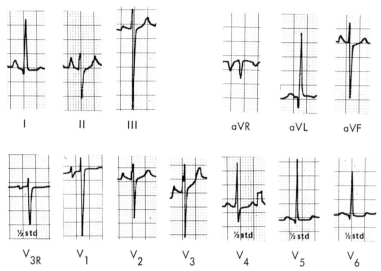

Fig. 9–6. — Electrocardiogram of a patient with tricuspid atresia. The salient features are a tall P wave in II — right atrial hypertrophy. The deep S wave in V_1 and tall R waves in $V_{5, 6}$ are interpretable as left ventricular hypertrophy. The negative P wave in V_{3R} suggests left atrial hypertrophy. The dominant R_I and S_{III} is left axis deviation.

The arrows represent alteration in the size of a chamber or a vessel as follows:

↑ Increased
↓ Decreased

This information can logically be translated to the x-ray, where one would expect to find an enlarged right atrium, left atrium, left ventricle and aorta. The vascular markings to the lungs would be diminished (Fig. 9–5). The electrocardiogram would also show right atrial, left atrial and left ventricular hypertrophy. The axis will be leftward (Fig. 9–6).

CLINICAL APPLICATION

This is as clear a left-sided lesion as exists. The physical findings will quite clearly relate to the anatomy as described. The patient will present cyanotic and usually deeply so. The precordium will not be particularly prominent but there may be a left ventricular thrust. The first sound will be single, there being an absence of its tricuspid portion. The second sound usually will be single but there may be a semblance of pulmonary component if there is a stenotic pulmonary valve (one of the rarer varieties). The nature of the murmur is variable at best. One might hear a diastolic murmur due to flow across the mitral valve. If the ventricular septal defect is significant, a holosystolic murmur may present at the lower left sternal border. If pulmonary stenosis is present, an ejection murmur from flow through the stenotic valve can be anticipated. Lastly and most commonly, no murmur at all may be heard.

Characteristically, the patient with this lesion presents in early infancy with cyanosis. Hypoxic spells are common and right heart failure may occur also. The diagnosis can be suspected on the basis of the chest x-ray showing diminished vascular markings and the electrocardiogram showing left axis deviation and

Fig. 9−7.−Echocardiograms of a normal newborn (**A**) and a patient with tricuspid atresia (**B**). Note the relatively small right ventricle and very large left ventricle in the patient with tricuspid atresia. *ECG* = electrocardiogram, *CW* = chest wall, *RV* = right ventricle, *S* = septum, *LV* = left ventricle, *MV* = mitral valve. (Modified from Meyer, R. A., and Kaplan, S.: Prog. Cardiovasc. Dis. 15:341, 1973.)

pure left ventricular hypertrophy. An echocardiogram can be helpful in demonstrating a diminutive right ventricular chamber and no tricuspid valve (Fig. 9–7). The diagnosis can be confirmed with cardiac catheterization, during which elevated pressures in both atria, inability to enter the right ventricle and decreased saturation in the left atrium, left ventricle and systemic artery will be found (Table 9–1). The diagnosis is firmly established with the use of angiocardiography, for the flow of dye goes from the right atrium to the left atrium, to the left ventricle and out the aorta. A radiolucent area replaces the expected location of the right ventricle (Figs. 9–8 and 9–9). Pulmonary flow is established through either a ductus arteriosus, bronchial circulation or, when present, a small ventricular septal defect that leads to the pulmonary artery.

It should be mentioned that types IC and IIC (see classification above), each of which has a large ventricular septal defect

TABLE 9–1.—IDEALIZED CARDIAC CATHETERIZATION DATA
IN A PATIENT WITH TRICUSPID ATRESIA*

SITE	PRESSURE (mm Hg)		OXYGEN SATURATION (%)	
	Normal	Patient	Normal	Patient
Superior vena cava			70	41
Inferior vena cava			74	45
Right atrium	a = 5 v = 3 m = 4	a = 12 v = 8 m = 7	72	45
Right ventricle	25/2	Not entered	72	Not entered
Main pulmonary artery	25/12	Not entered	72	Not entered
Left atrium	a = 5 v = 7 m = 6	a = 10 v = 8 m = 7	97	58
Left ventricle	105/5	105/5	97	58
Systemic artery	105/60	105/60	97	58
Pulmonary vein	a = 5 v = 7 m = 7	a = 10 v = 8 m = 8	97	97

*The salient features are elevated pressures in the right and left atria and failure to enter the right ventricle. There is a decrease in the oxygen saturation in the left atrium as compared to the pulmonary veins (this suggests a right-to-left shunt across the atrial septum). Peripheral saturation is also diminished.

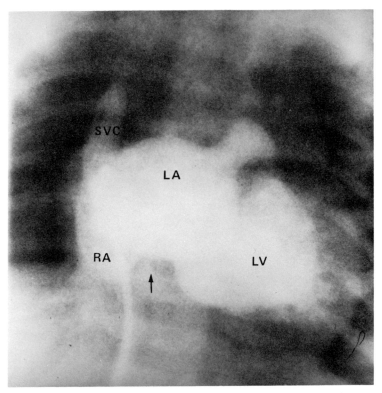

Fig. 9–8. — Enlargement of a single frame from a cineangiocardiogram of a patient with tricuspid atresia. Note the right atrium, left atrium, left ventricle and superior vena cava. The arrow is pointing to the expected location of the right ventricle, which is not opacified. *RA* = right atrium, *LA* = left atrium, *LV* = left ventricle, *SVC* = superior vena cava.

without pulmonary stenosis, present in a different fashion. The increased pulmonary flow may result in left heart failure, and the clinical picture more closely resembles the findings in a patient with a ventricular septal defect but with mild cyanosis. The heart would be larger on x-ray and the vessels increased. The electrocardiogram would show more right ventricular hypertrophy than in the other types (not illustrated).

Fig. 9–9. – Enlargement of a single frame from a cineangiocardiogram of a patient with tricuspid atresia, taken slightly later in systole than Figure 9–8. Note the appearance of the aorta. The right ventricular area *(arrow)* is narrowed but persists. *RA* = right atrium, *LV* = left ventricle, *Ao* = aorta.

DIFFERENTIAL DIAGNOSIS

Initially, the patient with tricuspid atresia must be differentiated from one having transposition of the great arteries, truncus arteriosus, total anomalous pulmonary venous connection and tetralogy of Fallot. The presence of dominant left ventricular hypertrophy in the electrocardiogram will virtually eliminate all of these lesions from serious consideration.

The major lesion presenting confusion is pulmonary atresia with an intact ventricular septum and a normal tricuspid valve. Blood does pass through the tricuspid valve into the right ventricle but then refluxes back to the right atrium, to follow the circulation of the patient with tricuspid atresia. Pulmonary atresia can be suspected if there are right-sided forces in the electrocardiogram as shown by the presence of normal or right axis deviation and an R wave in V_1 and an S wave in $V_{5, 6}$.

PEARLS

1. There is no sex differentiation with this lesion.

2. Intense cyanosis in a newborn with left ventricular hypertrophy in the electrocardiogram strongly suggests the diagnosis.

3. Pulmonary atresia with intact ventricular septum should be ruled out because the therapy of the two lesions may differ.

4. Without surgical intervention, early death can be anticipated.

5. The recognition of cyanosis is enough indication to perform a heart catheterization with angiocardiography.

6. Remember that the risk of catheterization in the newborn is in the range of 5%. This should not be a deterrent to the study but rather a realism.

CHAPTER TEN

Transposition of the Great Arteries

EMBRYOLOGY

TOWARD the end of the third week and into the fourth, the common trunk is divided into the pulmonary artery and the aorta. This is accomplished by a caudad spiral growth of the truncoconal ridges (Fig. 10–1).

The mechanism behind this spiral growth is subject to several basic theories. The first suggests that the spiral motion of the

Fig. 10–1. – Diagrammatic representation of the division of the truncus arteriosus (**A**) into the aorta and the pulmonary artery (**C**). Panel **B** shows the septation and the spiral direction of the pulmonary artery and the aorta. *PA* = pulmonary artery, *Ao* = aorta.

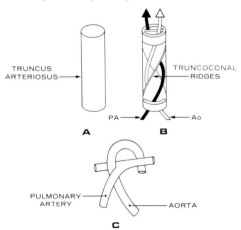

blood from each potential ventricular chamber into the truncus arteriosus causes the septum to assume a corresponding spiral direction. This would result in the left ventricle emptying its blood into a vessel that would become the aorta, and the right ventricle emptying its blood into a vessel that would become the pulmonary artery. A second theory suggests that as the bulbus cordis develops, it enlarges and rotates, carrying with it the truncoconal septum in such a way that the aorta will arise from the left ventricle and the pulmonary artery from the right ventricle. If there is disruption of either of these two mechanisms, the septum will grow in a straight caudad direction, disrupting the expected relationship between the great vessels and the ventricular chambers.

ANATOMY

By definition, when the great arteries are transposed, the aorta will arise from the anterior ventricle. This being a right ventricle, it will have an infundibulum, and the aortic valve and its sinuses will sit on top of that infundibulum. The normal continuity between the aortic and mitral valve rings will be lost. The pulmonary artery will arise from the posterior ventricle. This being a left ventricle, it will not have an infundibulum, and the pulmonary valves will have been drawn down inferiorly and posteriorly, putting the pulmonary valve ring in continuity with the mitral valve ring. The root of the aorta, therefore, will be anterior, superior and rightward in its location whereas the root of the pulmonary artery will be posterior, inferior and leftward in its location (Fig. 10–2).

Although the basic embryologic error that results in transposition of the great arteries may leave the remainder of the heart totally intact, there can be coexisting lesions. The most commonly found additional defects are patent ductus arteriosus, ventricular septal defect, ventricular septal defect with subpulmonic stenosis and, much less commonly, any combination of the three. For the sake of simplicity, the remainder of this chapter will be devoted to discussing transposition of the great arteries as it occurs with an intact ventricular septum, with a ven-

Fig. 10–2. – Diagrammatic representation of the anatomy seen in a patient with transposition of the great arteries (**B**) as compared to the normal (**A**). (See text for explanation.) *IVC* = inferior vena cava, *SVC* = superior vena cava, *RA* = right atrium, *RV* = right ventricle, *LA* = left atrium, *LV* = left ventricle.

tricular septal defect or with a ventricular septal defect and subpulmonic stenosis.

TRANSPOSITION OF THE GREAT ARTERIES WITH INTACT VENTRICULAR SEPTUM

Hemodynamics

The patient with transposition of the great arteries with an intact ventricular septum has two parallel circuits and can be depicted conceptually in the mnemonic

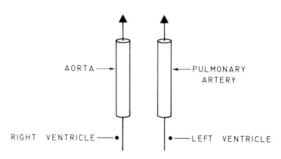

The arrows represent the blood flow from each ventricle into its respective great vessel. It should be noted that the right ventricle leads to the aorta and the left ventricle to the pulmonary artery. Although, for diagrammatic purposes, the great vessels are shown side by side, it must be remembered that in the patient they actually relate to each other in an anteroposterior direction. If the blood flow is followed with the mnemonic in mind, the effect on the various chambers and vessels of the heart can be demonstrated by the following diagram:

RIGHT ATRIUM ↑   LEFT ATRIUM →
RIGHT VENTRICLE ↑   LEFT VENTRICLE →
AORTA →   MAIN PULMONARY ARTERY →
                                   PULMONARY VESSELS ↑

The arrows represent alteration in the size of a chamber or a vessel as follows:

→ Unchanged
↑ Increased

Fig. 10–3.—Chest roentgenograms of an infant with transposition of the great arteries. Note the slightly enlarged right atrium and right ventricle. The mediastinum is narrow. The pulmonary vessels are somewhat increased. The over-all cardiac size is slightly larger than normal. *RA* = right atrium, *RV* = right ventricle, *M* = mediastinum, *PV* = pulmonary vessels.

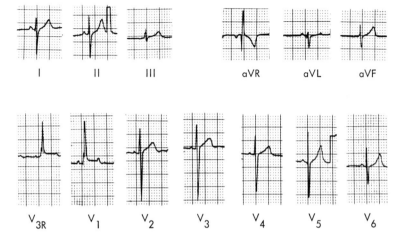

Fig. 10–4.—Electrocardiogram of an infant with transposition of the great arteries. The salient features are the dominant S_I and R_{III}—right axis deviation. There is also a dominant R wave in V_1 and S wave in $V_{5, 6}$, which is interpretable as right ventricular hypertrophy. The T wave in V_1 is also upright.

This information can be translated to the chest x-ray, where one would expect cardiomegaly, with an enlarged right atrium and right ventricle. Because the great vessels relate in an antero-posterior direction, the mediastinum will be narrow. The blood flow to the lungs normally is increased and therefore the vascular markings would be increased (Fig. 10–3). The electrocardiogram would show right ventricular hypertrophy and perhaps right atrial hypertrophy (Fig. 10–4).

Clinical Application

It must be recalled that the patient essentially has two independent parallel circuits and that life is dependent on some intermixing of those two circuits. This occurs through the foramen ovale and the ductus arteriosus. Physiologic closure of both would result in sudden death. Depending on the degree of intermixing through the ductus arteriosus and the foramen ovale, the infant will be either minimally cyanotic or intensely blue. The bidirectional flow is dependent on subtle changes in systemic and pulmonary resistances and usually is in such low volume as not to cause a murmur. Even though there are two great vessels and two sets of valves, the common auscultatory finding is that of a single intensified second sound. This usually represents closure of the aortic valve, which is close to the chest wall.

The diagnosis can be suspected in a male infant who has minimal to moderate cyanosis, no significant murmurs and a single second sound. The chest x-ray will show cardiomegaly, a narrow mediastinum and increased vascular markings. The electrocardiogram will show right ventricular hypertrophy and possibly right atrial hypertrophy. The diagnosis can be confirmed with cardiac catheterization, which will demonstrate peripheral desaturation, systemic pressures in the right ventricle, the aorta arising from the right ventricle and in the pulmonary artery arising from the left ventricle (Table 10–1). Cineangiocardiography will show the great vessel relationship (Figs. 10–5 and 10–6).

Parenthetically, it should be commented that frequently in the first day of life, the x-ray and electrocardiogram will not have

TABLE 10–1.—IDEALIZED CARDIAC CATHETERIZATION DATA
IN AN INFANT WITH TRANSPOSITION OF THE GREAT ARTERIES
AND INTACT VENTRICULAR SEPTUM*

SITE	PRESSURE (mm Hg)		OXYGEN SATURATION (%)	
	Normal	Patient	Normal	Patient
Superior vena cava			70	48
Inferior vena cava			74	52
Right atrium	a = 5 v = 4 m = 4	a = 5 v = 4 m = 4	72	50
Right ventricle	25/2	65/2	72	50
Aorta	65/40	65/40	97	50
Left atrium	a = 5 v = 7 m = 6	a = 5 v = 7 m = 6	97	97
Left ventricle	65/2	25/2	97	97
Main pulmonary artery	25/12	25/12	72	97

*The salient feature is decreased oxygen saturation in the right side of the heart as well as the aorta. The pressures in the right ventricle are systemic in height whereas those in the left ventricle and the main pulmonary artery are low. The order of the sites indicates that the aorta arises from the right ventricle and the main pulmonary artery from the left ventricle.

A   **B**

Fig. 10–5.—Enlargements of two 35-mm cineangiocardiographic frames in a patient with transposition of the great arteries. Note that the aorta arises from the right ventricle and that the main pulmonary artery fills from the ductus arteriosus. *C* = catheter, *RV* = right ventricle, *Ao* = aorta, *DA* = ductus arteriosus, *MPA* = main pulmonary artery. Panel **A**, anteroposterior projection. Panel **B**, lateral projection.

Fig. 10–6.—Enlargements of two 35-mm cineangiocardiographic frames in a patient with transposition of the great arteries. Note that the main pulmonary artery arises from the left ventricle. *C* = catheter, *LV* = left ventricle, *MPA* = main pulmonary artery, *LAa* = left atrial appendage. Panel **A**, anteroposterior projection. Panel **B**, lateral projection.

A   **B**

assumed the classic findings as discussed above. They may be very close to normal, making the diagnosis much more elusive. Within a few short days, however, if an index of suspicion is maintained, evidence for the existence of congenital heart disease will mount and cardiac catheterization will permit the establishment of an accurate diagnosis.

TRANSPOSITION OF THE GREAT ARTERIES WITH VENTRICULAR SEPTAL DEFECT

Hemodynamics

This combination of defects can be demonstrated in the mnemonic

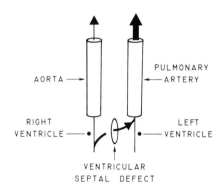

The arrows represent the blood flow from each ventricle into its respective great vessel plus right-to-left flow through the ventricular septal defect. If the blood flow is followed with mnemonic in mind, the effect on the various chambers and vessels of the heart can be demonstrated by the following diagram:

RIGHT ATRIUM → ↑	LEFT ATRIUM → ↑
RIGHT VENTRICLE ↑	LEFT VENTRICLE → ↑
AORTA →	MAIN PULMONARY ARTERY → ↑
	PULMONARY VESSELS ↑

The arrows represent changes in the size of a chamber or a vessel as follows:

→ Unchanged
↑ Increased

Translated to the chest x-ray, one would expect to find a normal or slightly enlarged right atrium, an enlarged right ventricle and a normal to enlarged left atrium and left ventricle. Because the great vessels relate in an anteroposterior direction, the mediastinum would be narrow. The pulmonary vascular markings would be increased. These findings are so similar to those in a patient with an intact ventricular septum that Figure 10–3 remains representative. The electrocardiogram would be expected to show biventricular hypertrophy. The degree of left ventricular hypertrophy is dependent on the size of the ventricular septal defect and the degree of pulmonary vascular resistance. Despite these theoretic and practical statements, right ventricular hypertrophy generally is seen (see Fig. 10–4).

Clinical Application

Because the pulmonary resistance at birth generally is equal to the systemic resistance, there is little flow across the ventricular septal defect. The patient with transposition of the great arteries with ventricular septal defect, therefore, may be indistinguishable from one without a ventricular septal defect. It is only after there is some drop in pulmonary resistance through natural maturation that the clinical picture will change. As this resistance drops, shunting can take place through the defect. In this instance, because the left ventricle relates to the pulmonary circuit, it will have the lower pressure and the shunting will be from the right ventricle to the left ventricle. There then will occur a holosystolic murmur at the fourth interspace to the left of the sternum and, if loud enough, it will be accompanied by a thrill. The flow through the ventricular septal defect will pass through the pulmonary vessels and be returned to the left atrium. This increased volume will enlarge the size of the atrium, stretch the foramen ovale and permit the shunting of oxygenated blood into the right atrium. It should be apparent that this combination of anatomic and physiologic communications will permit the delivery of venous blood to the lungs and oxygenated blood to the body. It also must be stated that the increased flow of blood under an increased head of pressure to the pulmonary circuit places the lung at risk for the development of pulmonary vascular disease. The remainder of the examination will be similar to that in a patient with an intact ventricular septum and will not be repeated here. This diagnosis can be suspected in a male infant who has findings suggestive of transposition of the great arteries but who has holosystolic murmur at the fourth interspace to the left of the sternum. The chest x-ray would show cardiomegaly, a narrow mediastinum and increased vascular markings, and the electrocardiogram would show dominant right ventricular hypertrophy. Cardiac catheterization will demonstrate peripheral desaturation, systemic pressures in the right ventricle, the aorta arising from the right ventricle and, more specifically, evidence of left-to-right shunting at the atrial level and right-to-left shunting at the ventricular level. Cineangiocardiography would demonstrate the ventricular septal defect and the great vessel abnormality.

TRANSPOSITION OF THE GREAT ARTERIES WITH VENTRICULAR SEPTAL DEFECT AND SUBPULMONIC STENOSIS

Hemodynamics

The patient with this combination of defects has markedly diminished blood flow to the lungs and can be depicted in the mnemonic

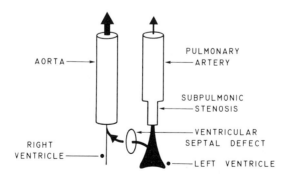

The arrows represent the blood flow from each ventricle into its respective great vessel. The smaller arrow leaving the pulmonary artery suggests the diminished blood flow to the lungs. The narrowed part of the pulmonary artery represents the subpulmonic stenosis. The heavy base of the arrow below the pulmonary artery suggests the increased pressure in the left ventricle. The shunting through the ventricular septal defect is shown as a heavy arrow passing through it and entering the aorta, with a resultant greater flow through the aorta, as shown by the heavier arrow leaving that great vessel. If the blood flow is followed with the mnemonic in mind, the effect on the various chambers and vessels of the heart can be demonstrated by the following diagram:

RIGHT ATRIUM ↑	LEFT ATRIUM →
RIGHT VENTRICLE ↑	LEFT VENTRICLE ↑
AORTA →	MAIN PULMONARY ARTERY → ↓
	PULMONARY VESSELS ↓

The arrows represent the effect on the heart and great vessels as follows:

→ Unchanged
↑ Increased
↓ Decreased

These changes can be translated to the chest x-ray, where one would expect to find cardiomegaly with right atrial and biventricular enlargement. The mediastinum would be narrow because of the anteroposterior relationship of the great vessels. The pulmonary vascular markings would be diminished. Aside from the diminished pulmonary vascular markings, the findings are similar enough to those seen in a patient with an intact ventricular septum to permit Figure 10-3 to be representative. Although theoretically the electrocardiogram should show biventricular hypertrophy, the usual finding is only right ventricular hypertrophy (see Fig. 10-4).

Clinical Application

With this combination, the subpulmonic stenosis creates a higher resistance to pulmonary flow than systemic flow, thus permitting the delivery of more oxygenated blood from the left ventricle through the ventricular septal defect to the aorta. One might then expect the patient to become less cyanotic. However, as the pulmonary stenosis becomes more severe, the patient actually becomes more cyanotic. With the increase in pulmonary stenosis, the resistance of flow to the lungs increases and there is a diminution in pulmonary flow. This results in a decrease in left atrial pressure, which, with the consistently elevated right atrial pressure, will cause a right-to-left shunt at the level of the atria. The mixing of poorly oxygenated systemic venous blood with the well-oxygenated pulmonary venous blood will result in an over-all diminished saturation of blood delivered to the left ventricle. The cycle repeats itself to such a degree that blood leaving the left ventricle through the ventricular septal defect to the aorta becomes progressively lower in saturation.

The basic physical findings will be similar to those in any other patient with transposition of the great arteries. There will be, in addition, a systolic ejection murmur high along the left sternal border representing flow through the subpulmonic stenosis.

The diagnosis can be suspected in an infant who has findings suggestive of transposition of the great arteries but who is more cyanotic, has an ejection systolic murmur along the left sternal border, a chest x-ray with cardiomegaly, a narrow mediastinum and decreased vascular markings and an electrocardiogram with dominant right ventricular hypertrophy. Cardiac catheterization will demonstrate peripheral desaturation, systemic pressures in both ventricles, the origin of the aorta from the right ventricle, the origin of the pulmonary artery from the left ventricle and, if entered, low pressures in the pulmonary artery. Cineangiocardiography would identify the ventricular septal defect, the subpulmonic stenosis and the great vessel relationship.

DIFFERENTIAL DIAGNOSIS

The patient with transposition of the great arteries must be differentiated from one having truncus arteriosus, total anomalous pulmonary venous connection, tricuspid atresia and, rarely, tetralogy of Fallot (note that all of these lesions begin with the letter t). Each of these lesions is discussed in detail in its respective chapter.

The patient with truncus arteriosus is similar in that cyanosis appears at about the same time and the second sound is single, but differs in that murmurs are rather consistently present and frequently continuous in character, the chest x-ray shows a wide mediastinum and cardiomegaly and the electrocardiogram shows biventricular hypertrophy. Cardiac catheterization will demonstrate the single great artery, completing the differential.

The patient with total anomalous pulmonary venous connection with obstruction will be easily differentiated on the basis of a small heart on x-ray. One without obstruction will have a well-split second sound, an ejection systolic murmur along the left sternal border and cardiomegaly on x-ray.

The patient with tricuspid atresia will also be cyanotic, but the presence of left axis deviation and left ventricular hypertrophy on the electrocardiogram will quickly make the differential clear.

The patient with tetralogy of Fallot, although included in the differential on the basis of cyanosis, is easily differentiated. The cyanosis occurs later in life, murmurs are heard consistently and the chest x-ray shows diminished vascular markings and a boot-shaped heart and lacks a narrow mediastinum.

PEARLS

1. Transposition of the great arteries is more common in males than in females.

2. The cyanosis may be quite subtle.

3. The diagnosis on the first day of life may be extremely difficult and a high index of suspicion must persist.

4. The birth weight of patients with transposition of the great arteries usually is normal or greater than normal.

CHAPTER ELEVEN
Truncus Arteriosus

EMBRYOLOGY

TOWARD the end of the third week and into the fourth, the common trunk normally is divided into the pulmonary artery and the aorta. This is accomplished by the development of the truncoconal ridges, which grow caudad in a spiral fashion, resulting in the posterolateral takeoff of the aorta and the anteromedial takeoff of the pulmonary artery (Fig. 11 – 1). This septum fuses with the bulbar ridges, which, in turn, participate with the endocardial cushions and membranous proliferation from the ventricular septum to form the definitive closure of the interventricular septum (Fig. 11 – 2).

Fig. 11–1. – Diagrammatic representation of the division of the truncus arteriosus (**A**) into the aorta and the pulmonary artery (**C**). Panel **B** shows the septation and the spiral direction of the pulmonary artery and the aorta. *PA* = pulmonary artery, *Ao* = aorta.

Fig. 11–2. – Diagrammatic representation of the final fusion of the ventricular septum and its relationship to the bulbar ridges.

ANATOMY

If the septation of the common trunk fails to take place, a single great vessel persists, which receives blood from both the left and right ventricles. Since the truncal septum participates in the final closure of the ventricular septum, there must be a ventricu-

Fig. 11–3. – Classification of truncus arteriosus. **A,** type I, **B,** type II, **C,** type III, **D,** type IV. (See text for explanation.)

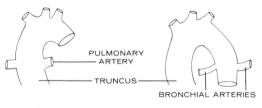

lar septal defect in conjunction with the common trunk (one of the rare "musts" in medicine). As in most of pediatric cardiology, variations on the theme have occurred and truncus arteriosus has been subdivided into four basic anatomic varieties. Type I (Fig. 11–3, *A*) has a common trunk arising from the heart and a partial septation of that trunk giving rise to the dominant aorta and the right and left pulmonary arteries as shown. Type II (Fig. 11–3, *B*) has pulmonary arteries that arise from the posterior surface of the common trunk. Type III (Fig. 11–3, *C*) has pulmonary arteries arising from the lateral walls of the common trunk. Type IV (Fig. 11–3, *D*) has no pulmonary arteries at al but rather bronchial arteries arising from the descending aorta.

HEMODYNAMICS

Regardless of the anatomic variety present, the patient with a truncus arteriosus has a common outlet for both right and left ventricular output. The blood flow to the lungs, however, will vary from increased to diminished, depending on the specific anatomic variety present. The over-all concept is shown in the mnemonic

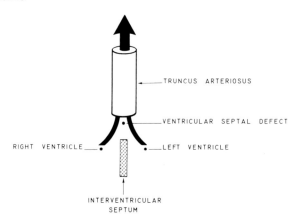

The arrows represent blood flow from each ventricle into the common trunk.

In the first three types of truncus arteriosus, pulmonary arteries are present and arise in one way or another from the common trunk. If this is kept in mind and the flow followed, the effect on the heart can be demonstrated by the following diagram:

RIGHT ATRIUM →   LEFT ATRIUM →
RIGHT VENTRICLE ↑   LEFT VENTRICLE ↑
BRANCH PULMONARY ARTERIES ↑   TRUNK ↑
PULMONARY VESSELS ↑

The arrows represent alteration in the size of a chamber or a vessel as follows:

→ Unchanged
↑ Increased

This information can be translated to the chest x-ray, where one would expect cardiomegaly, biventricular enlargement and a wide mediastinum. The pulmonary arteries frequently arise in a more superior location from the trunk and this may be seen on the x-ray. The vascular markings would be increased (Fig. 11–

Fig. 11–4.—Chest roentgenograms of a 1-year-old patient with type II truncus arteriosus. Note the cardiomegaly, wide mediastinum due to the large trunk, the enlarged right atrium, right ventricle and left ventricle. The pulmonary vessels are increased. *T* = trunk, *RA* = right atrium, *RV* = right ventricle, *LV* = left ventricle, *PV* = pulmonary vessels.

4). The electrocardiogram would show biventricular hypertrophy (Fig. 11–5).

In the fourth type of truncus arteriosus, no pulmonary artery is present and pulmonary circulation is through dilated bronchial arteries. If this is kept in mind, the flow as represented in the mnemonic would affect the heart as demonstrated in the following diagram:

RIGHT ATRIUM → ↑	LEFT ATRIUM →
RIGHT VENTRICLE ↑	LEFT VENTRICLE →
PULMONARY ARTERIES ○	AORTA →
PULMONARY VESSELS ↓	

The arrows represent alteration in the size of a chamber or a vessel as follows:

→ Unchanged
↑ Increased
↓ Decreased
○ Absent

Fig. 11–5. — Electrocardiogram of a 1-year-old patient with type II truncus arteriosus showing combined ventricular hypertrophy. The salient features are a dominant R wave in leads V_1 and $V_{5,6}$ and tall complexes in leads $V_{2,3,4}$.

Fig. 11–6. – Chest roentgenograms of a 1-year-old patient with type IV truncus arteriosus. The salient features are enlargement of the right atrium and right ventricle and diminished pulmonary vessels. *RA* = right atrium, *RV* = right ventricle, *PV* = pulmonary vessels.

Fig. 11–7. – Electrocardiograms of a 1-year-old patient with type IV truncus arteriosus. The salient features are the dominant S_1 and R_{III} – right axis deviation. There also is a dominant R wave in V_1 and S wave in $V_{5,6}$, which is interpretable as right ventricular hypertrophy. The T wave in V_1 is also upright.

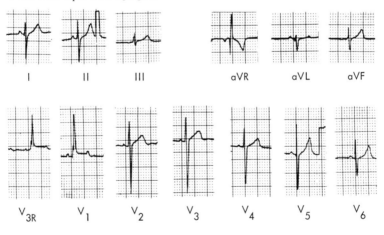

Once more translating this to the chest x-ray, one would expect to find right ventricular enlargement, an absence of the pulmonary artery bulge on the left border of the heart and very diminished pulmonary vessels (Fig. 11–6). The electrocardiogram would show dominant right ventricular hypertrophy (Fig. 11–7).

CLINICAL APPLICATION

Although each anatomic variation of truncus arteriosus will have subtle differences, there is sufficient similarity to permit presenting the entire panorama under a single subtitle noting the differences rather than going to the extent of totally separate presentations.

Because of the large dilated trunk, the onset of systole may be introduced with an ejection click. This will be followed by a systolic murmur, more ejection in quality than anything else and varying in intensity from grade II/VI to, rarely, grade IV/VI. It is heard at about the fourth interspace to the left of the sternum. It may well transmit along the great vessels of the aorta and

TABLE 11–1.—IDEALIZED CARDIAC CATHETERIZATION DATA IN A 1-YEAR-OLD PATIENT WITH TYPE II TRUNCUS ARTERIOSUS*

SITE	PRESSURE (mm Hg)		OXYGEN SATURATION (%)	
	Normal	Patient	Normal	Patient
Superior vena cava			70	60
Inferior vena cava			74	68
Right atrium	a = 5 v = 3 m = 4	a = 9 v = 6 m = 5	72	64
Right ventricle	25/2	100/8	72	64
Pulmonary artery	25/2	100/40	72	76
Left atrium	a = 5 v = 7 m = 6	a = 7 v = 12 m = 10	97	97
Left ventricle	100/5	100/4	97	97
Aorta (trunk)	100/55	100/55	97	76

*The salient features are slightly elevated pressures in the right atrium, systemic pressures in the right ventricle and the pulmonary artery and desaturation in the aorta and the pulmonary artery.

much less frequently into the pulmonary arteries. At times, a continuous murmur can be heard on the anterior chest. The diastolic component may be related to flow into the pulmonary arteries during the diastolic phase of the cardiac cycle. Because there is a single set of leaflets — three or four in number — and not two separate sets of semilunar valves, the second sound can be

Fig. 11–8.—An enlargement of a single 35-mm frame taken from a cineangiocardiogram performed on a 1-year-old patient with type II truncus arteriosus. The tip of the catheter is in the right ventricle. The salient features are the enlarged trunk and the presence of a right pulmonary artery and a left pulmonary artery, which arise from the posterior aspect of the trunk. C = catheter, RV = right ventricle, T = trunk, RPA = right pulmonary artery, LPA = left pulmonary artery.

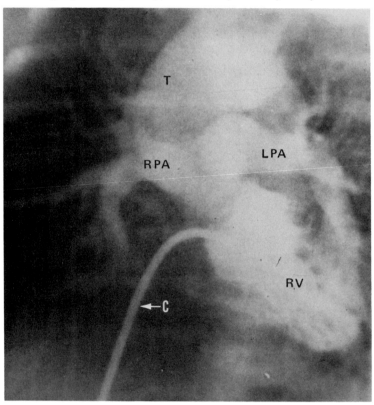

anticipated to be single. This is a very consistent finding. The blood flow into the lungs will be variable, depending on the pulmonary resistance. If this flow happens to be significant, the return to the left atrium may result in a mid-diastolic filling sound as it passes across the mitral valve. Also, continuous murmurs may be heard across the back as well as the anterior chest due to bronchial flow.

The patient with truncus arteriosus is consistently cyanotic. However, the degree of cyanosis may vary from minimal (when there is adequate pulmonary flow) to intense (when the flow is through small bronchial arteries). If there is significant pulmonary flow (types I, II and III), the burden on the left side of the heart can result in early congestive heart failure. The usual symptoms of cough and signs of tachypnea with dyspnea, tachycardia and hepatomegaly will be seen. Cardiac catheterization almost always will be required and will show a decrease in oxygen saturation on the right side of the heart and a further decrease in the aorta. The pressures in the right ventricle and, if entered, the pulmonary artery will be systemic in height. There also is minimal elevation of both the right and left atrial pressures (Table 11 – 1). Cineangiocardiography would demonstrate

TABLE 11–2.—IDEALIZED CARDIAC CATHETERIZATION DATA IN A 1-YEAR-OLD PATIENT WITH TYPE IV TRUNCUS ARTERIOSUS*

SITE	PRESSURE (mm Hg)		OXYGEN SATURATION (%)	
	Normal	Patient	Normal	Patient
Superior vena cava			70	43
Inferior vena cava			74	49
Right atrium	a = 5 v = 3 m = 4	a = 12 v = 7 m = 9	72	45
Right ventricle	25/2	100/5	72	45
Main pulmonary artery	25/12	Not entered	72	Not entered
Left atrium	a = 5 v = 7 m = 6	a = 5 v = 7 m = 6	97	97
Left ventricle	100/5	100/5	97	97
Aorta (trunk)	100/55	100/55	97	65

*The salient features are an increase in pressure in the right atrium, systemic pressures in the right ventricle, the inability to enter a pulmonary artery, desaturation in the right atrium and ventricle and desaturation in the aorta.

the large common trunk and the origin of the pulmonary arteries (Fig. 11 – 8).

If there is insufficient pulmonary flow (type IV), the patient tends not to go into heart failure but rather to be exposed to the risks of severe hypoxia. These are acidosis and, more threateningly, hypoxic spells. During cardiac catheterization, the pulmonary artery cannot be entered and systemic pressures in the right ventricle and systemic desaturations will be found (Table 11 – 2). Angiocardiography will confirm the absence of a main pulmonary artery and the presence of some form of bronchial circulation (Fig. 11 – 9).

Fig. 11 – 9. – An enlargement of a single 35-mm frame taken from a cineangiocardiogram performed on a 1-year-old patient with type IV truncus arteriosus. The tip of the catheter is in the ascending trunk. The salient features are the presence of a bronchial artery arising from the descending aorta and the filling of the right pulmonary artery from the bronchial artery. C = catheter, T = trunk, BA = bronchial artery, Ao = aorta, RPA = right pulmonary artery.

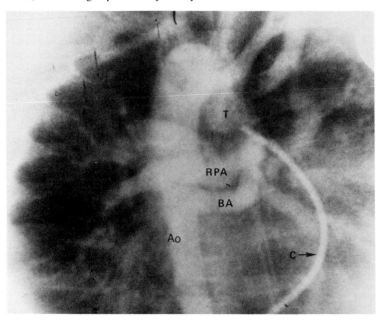

The diagnosis of the first three types of truncus arteriosus can be suspected in an infant who is cyanotic, with a single second sound, murmurs varying from minimal to continuous, the chest x-ray showing cardiomegaly, displaced pulmonary arteries and increased vascular markings and an electrocardiogram showing combined ventricular hypertrophy. The patient with the fourth type will be a deeper blue, have less of a murmur, a single second sound, an x-ray with diminished vascular markings and an electrocardiogram showing right ventricular hypertrophy.

DIFFERENTIAL DIAGNOSIS

The patient with truncus arteriosus must be differentiated from one having transposition of the great arteries, total anomalous pulmonary venous connection, tricuspid atresia and tetralogy of Fallot (note that all of these lesions begin with the letter t). Each of them is discussed in detail in its respective chapter.

The patient with transposition of the great arteries is similar in that the cyanosis appears early in infancy and the second sound is single, but differs in that murmurs generally are absent and the chest x-ray shows a narrow mediastinum with cardiomegaly and the electrocardiogram shows right ventricular hypertrophy. Cardiac catheterization will demonstrate the transposed great arteries.

The patient with total anomalous pulmonary venous connection with obstruction will be easily differentiated on the basis of a small heart on x-ray. One without obstruction will have a well-split second sound, an ejection systolic murmur along the left sternal border, cardiomegaly on x-ray, not presented clinically until after infancy. The patient with tricuspid atresia will only momentarily be considered on the basis of cyanosis. The presence of dominant left ventricular hypertrophy on the electrocardiogram will quickly make the differential clear.

The patient with tetralogy of Fallot will be very reminiscent of the patient with type IV truncus arteriosus. Cardiac catheterization almost certainly will be required to show the presence of a pulmonary artery arising from the right ventricle in tetralogy of

Fallot as compared to the total absence of a pulmonary artery in truncus arteriosus.

PEARLS

1. Splitting of the second sound rules out truncus arteriosus.
2. There is no sex difference.
3. A right aortic arch is seen frequently.

CHAPTER TWELVE
Ebstein's Anomaly

EMBRYOLOGY

AT ABOUT the fifth week of gestation there is a blending of the anterior endocardial cushion, the posterior endocardial cushion, a portion of the interventricular septum and the ventricular muscle itself to form the right atrioventricular canal and subsequently the valve, known as the tricuspid valve (Figs. 12–1 and 12–2). The papillary muscles and chordae tendineae arise from careful sculpturing of the ventricular muscle (Fig. 12–3).

As the leaflets and chordae tendineae develop, so does the conduction system. This specialized muscle with the capability of transmitting impulses passes between the right atrium and the right ventricle. The AV node is located in the lower portion of the right atrium near the inferior vena cava and the coronary sinus. The bundle of His passes adjacent to the tricuspid valve

Fig. 12–1. – Schematic representation of the common atrioventricular canal developing into a right and a left canal. **A,** 30 days; **B,** 33 days; **C,** 35 days. (See text for explanation.) (Modified from Moss, A. J., and Adams, F. H. [eds.]: *Heart Disease in Infants, Children and Adolescents* [Baltimore: The Williams & Wilkins Company, 1968], p. 17.)

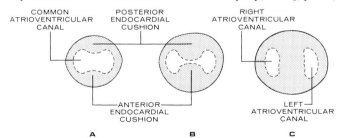

COMMON ATRIOVENTRICULAR CANAL

POSTERIOR ENDOCARDIAL CUSHION

RIGHT ATRIOVENTRICULAR CANAL

ANTERIOR ENDOCARDIAL CUSHION

LEFT ATRIOVENTRICULAR CANAL

A   B   C

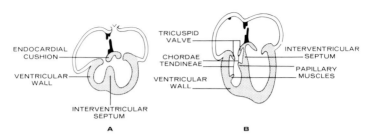

Fig. 12–2. – Schematic representation of the formation of the tricuspid valve. (See text for explanation.) Identification of left-sided structures has been omitted intentionally. **A,** 37 days; **B,** newborn. (Modified from Moss, A. J., and Adams, F. H. [eds.]: *Heart Disease in Infants, Children and Adolescents* [Baltimore: The Williams & Wilkins Company, 1968], p. 16.)

ring toward the interventricular septum, where it divides into right and left branches, which course along the respective sides of the right and left ventricles.

ANATOMY

If there is disruption of the above mechanism, the tricuspid valve annulus may be displaced downward, incorporating part of the normal right ventricle into the right atrium. The chordae

Fig. 12–3. – Schematic representation of the formation of the atrioventricular valves and their chordae tendineae and papillary muscles. (See text for explanation.) **A** and **B,** progressive stages of development. (Modified from Moss, A. J., and Adams, F. H. [eds.]: *Heart Disease in Infants, Children and Adolescents* [Baltimore: The Williams & Wilkins Company, 1968], p. 19.)

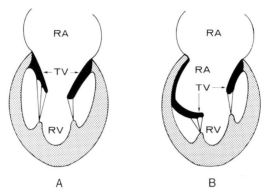

Fig. 12–4. – Diagrammatic representation of the anatomic appearance of the tricuspid valve in Ebstein's anomaly. Panel **A** shows the normal insertion of the tricuspid valve. Panel **B** shows the displacement of one leaflet of the tricuspid valve. Note the very small right ventricle and very large right atrium. *RA* = right atrium, *TV* = tricuspid valve, *RV* = right ventricle.

tendineae will be foreshortened and the total result is this anomaly, in which the right atrium is exceptionally large, the right ventricle particularly small and the tricuspid valve potentially or actually insufficient (Fig. 12–4). Errors in developmental patterns can also affect the conduction system. Incomplete disruption of the right-sided bundle can occur, leading to right bundle-branch block. An anomalous pathway across the tricuspid annulus can develop, resulting in the Wolff-Parkinson-White syndrome.

HEMODYNAMICS

The patient with Ebstein's anomaly of the tricuspid valve has an exceptionally dilated right atrium, which may secondarily stretch the atrial septum, rendering the foramen ovale incompetent. In the face of tricuspid insufficiency or other circumstances in which right atrial pressure would have increased beyond that of left atrial pressure, right-to-left shunting through the interatrial septum can take place. This concept is depicted in the mnemonic

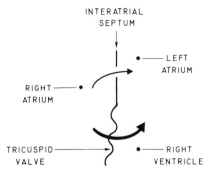

The mnemonic represents a long, patulous tricuspid valve with the interatrial septum above it. The thick arrow represents blood flowing through the tricuspid valve into the right ventricle in a normal fashion and the thin arrow represents blood flowing through the interatrial septum into the left atrium in an abnormal fashion. If the blood flow is followed with the mnemonic in

Fig. 12−5. − Chest roentgenograms of a child with Ebstein's anomaly. The salient features are a large right atrium and a prominent right ventricular outflow tract. *RA* = right atrium, *RVo* = right ventricular outflow tract.

mind, the effect on the heart and great vessels can be demonstrated by the following diagram:

RIGHT ATRIUM ↑   LEFT ATRIUM →
RIGHT VENTRICLE ↓   LEFT VENTRICLE →
MAIN PULMONARY ARTERY →   AORTA →
PULMONARY VESSELS → ↓

The arrows represent alteration in the size of a chamber or a vessel as follows:

→ Unchanged
↑ Increased
↓ Decreased

This information can be translated to the chest x-ray, where one would expect to find a very large right atrium, a small right ventricle but with a large outflow tract, which may be confusing, a normal main pulmonary artery and normal pulmonary vascular markings that are either normal or decreased (Fig. 12–5).

The electrocardiogram will show right atrial hypertrophy,

Fig. 12–6.—Electrocardiogram of a patient with Ebstein's anomaly showing right bundle-branch block. The salient features are the dominant S_I and R_{III}—right axis deviation—the wide QRS complex in all leads and the delayed notched R wave in lead V_{3R} and S wave in lead V_6. Note, however, that the R wave in lead V_1 is not very tall.

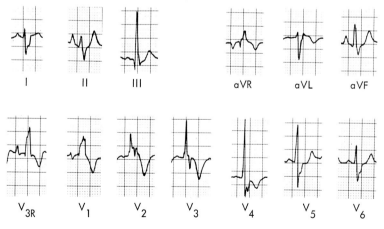

I   II   III   aVR   aVL   aVF

V_{3R} V_1 V_2 V_3 V_4 V_5 V_6

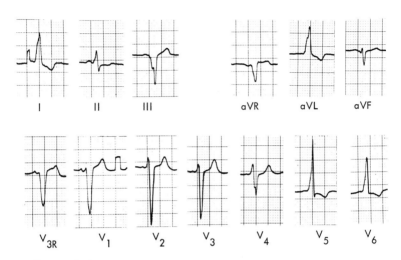

I   II   III   aVR   aVL   aVF

V$_{3R}$ V$_1$ V$_2$ V$_3$ V$_4$ V$_5$ V$_6$

all ½ standard

Fig. 12–7.—Electrocardiogram of a child with Ebstein's anomaly showing the Wolff-Parkinson-White syndrome. The salient features are a short P–R interval in all leads, a very wide QRS complex in all leads and the slurred initial component of the QRS in most leads—the delta wave.

absence of right ventricular hypertrophy and possibly left atrial and left ventricular hypertrophy. In addition, and very commonly indeed, will be the presence of conduction defects, such as right bundle-branch block (Fig. 12–6) and Wolff-Parkinson-White syndrome (Fig. 12–7).

CLINICAL APPLICATION

Unless the patient with Ebstein's anomaly of the tricuspid valve is subject to significant tricuspid insufficiency, he usually will grow to early childhood with insignificant symptoms. At that time, he may present with some diminution in exercise capability. Cyanosis may be apparent or so minimal as not to be visible. He will appear small to normal in size, with a chest that has a prominent left side. To palpation, the right atrial activity may be felt low in the chest to the right of the sternum, but a classic right ventricular heave should be absent. A left apical thrust may be palpable.

The rhythm of the heart to auscultation is unusual but characteristic. Although the mitral valve closes normally, the tricuspid valve closure generally is delayed and intensified. A prominent third heart sound is common due to filling of the right ventricle. Also, an atrial sound generally is present. Even though there are two bicuspid valves, the second sound usually is single. This conglomerate of events results in either a triple or a quadruple rhythm.

The most commonly heard murmur is that of tricuspid insufficiency. This early, medium-pitched, rather harsh systolic murmur is heard best at the location of the displaced tricuspid valve and therefore would be to the left of the sternum in the vicinity of the fourth or fifth intercostal space.

The cyanosis, when present, is a function of shunting across the atrial septum. Generally, it is only through an unguarded foramen ovale or rarely through a true ostium secundum defect. The quantity of blood flowing through the septum is related to the size of the right atrium and to the degree of tricuspid insufficiency. It should be clear, therefore, why the cyanosis may be minimal to modest. It also should be reasonably clear that the degree of left-sided involvement in terms of left atrial enlargement and left ventricular thrust would be dependent on the size of the intracardiac shunt.

If there is significant tricuspid insufficiency, the patient may get into trouble early in infancy. The diagnosis can be suspected in an infant who is in congestive heart failure with cyanosis, who has a large right atrium with diminished to normal pulmonary vascular markings in the chest x-ray and who may have conduction abnormalities in the electrocardiogram. The diagnosis can be strongly suspected in the catheterization laboratory by the demonstration of a large right atrium with elevated pressures and a small right ventricle with a low systolic pressure but a high diastolic pressure.

Right-to-left shunting at the level of the atria will be apparent. The diagnosis can be firmly confirmed with the use of intracardiac electrocardiography. With the catheter on the atrial side of

TABLE 12-1.—IDEALIZED CARDIAC CATHETERIZATION DATA
IN A CHILD WITH EBSTEIN'S ANOMALY*

SITE	PRESSURE (mm Hg)		OXYGEN SATURATION (%)	
	Normal	Patient	Normal	Patient
Superior vena cava			70	70
Inferior vena cava			74	74
Right atrium	a = 5 v = 3 m = 4	a = 14 v = 16 m = 14	72	72
Right ventricle	25/2	20/12	72	72
Main pulmonary artery	25/12	20/14	72	72
Pulmonary vein	a = 6 v = 8 m = 7	a = 7 v = 8 m = 8	97	97
Left atrium	a = 5 v = 7 m = 6	a = 6 v = 7 m = 7	97	85
Systemic artery	120/80	120/80	97	85

*The salient features are the elevated pressure in the right atrium and diminished systolic and elevated diastolic pressures in the right ventricle. In addition, the oxygen saturation in the left atrium is decreased when compared to the pulmonary vein. Peripheral saturation is decreased also.

the tricuspid valve, a ventricular pressure curve will be recorded and simultaneously an atrial electrocardiogram will be recorded (Table 12-1).

If the tricuspid insufficiency is negligible, the patient may well grow to early childhood before presenting with either a clinical panorama comparable to that in the infant or merely with rhythm disturbances as recognized in the electrocardiogram. The diagnosis once more can be confirmed in the catheterization laboratory, as just described.

DIFFERENTIAL DIAGNOSIS

The patient with Ebstein's anomaly must be differentiated from one with congenital tricuspid insufficiency but with normally inserted leaflets, one with pulmonary stenosis and right-to-left shunting through the foramen ovale and one with Uhl's disease.

The patient with congenital tricuspid insufficiency characteristically presents with congestive heart failure at birth. This may be most difficult to differentiate from Ebstein's anomaly but cardiac catheterization will be of help. With an intracardiac electro-cardiographic catheter placed near the tricuspid valve, an atrial pressure will be recorded along with an atrial electrocardiogram.

The patient with severe pulmonary stenosis characteristically has marked right ventricular hypertrophy in the electrocar-diogram, which should be sufficient to effect a differential.

Although the patient with Uhl's disease (underdeveloped right ventricle does have an effectual right ventricular chamber, it is dilated and has a parchment-thin wall. The tricuspid valve is normal in position, and cardiac catheterization should permit a differential diagnosis.

PEARLS

1. There is no sex preference.

2. The risk of cardiac catheterization is increased because of the high incidence of arrhythmias. However, this should not preclude the study when it is indicated.

CHAPTER THIRTEEN

Corrected Transposition of the Great Arteries

EMBRYOLOGY

AT ABOUT the third week of gestation, the primitive cardiac tube begins its earliest changes, which ultimately will transform it into a four-chambered heart. The tube is fixed in its attachments proximally and distally; and growing more rapidly than the peri-

Fig. 13–1.—Schematic representation of the development of the primitive cardiac tube into the definitive four-chambered heart. **A,** 18 days; **B,** 21 days; **C,** 23 days; **D,** 28 days. Note the initial rightward convex bending of the tube in panel **B.** RA = right atrium, LA = left atrium, RV = right ventricle, LV = left ventricle.

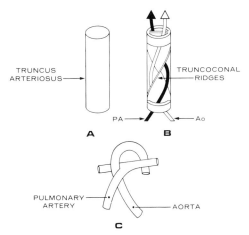

Fig. 13–2. – Diagrammatic representation of the division of the truncus arteriosus (**A**) into the aorta and the pulmonary artery (**C**). Panel **B** shows the septation and the spiral direction of the pulmonary artery and the aorta. PA = pulmonary artery, Ao = aorta.

cardial cavity, it folds on itself. The normal folding – called loop-ing – is convexly to the right, which results in the right ventricle being anterior and rightward and the left ventricle posterior and leftward. The atrioventricular valves passively follow their respective ventricles, so the three-leaflet tricuspid valve sits between the right atrium and the right ventricle and the two-leaflet mitral valve between the left atrium and the left ventricle (Fig. 13–1). A few days later, the common trunk is divided into two. The caudad spiral growth of the truncoconal ridges results in the origin of the aorta being posterior and leftward, arising from the left ventricle, and the origin of the pulmonary artery being anterior and rightward, arising from the right ventricle (Fig. 13–2).

ANATOMY

If, during embryologic growth, the loop does not twist to the right (commonly called *d* loop) but rather to the left (commonly

Fig. 13–3. – Diagrammatic representation of the anatomy of corrected transposition of the great arteries. Panel **A**, normal. Panel **B**, corrected transposition of the great arteries. Note that the pulmonary artery arises from the venous ventricle and the aorta from the arterial ventricle. SVC = superior vena cava, IVC = inferior vena cava, RA = right atrium, RV = right ventricle, PA = pulmonary artery, LA = left atrium, LV = left ventricle.

called *l* loop), the anatomic right ventricle will be displaced posteriorly and leftward, becoming the arterial ventricle, and the anatomic left ventricle will be displaced anteriorly and rightward, becoming the venous ventricle. The common trunk will be septated in a spiral nature but is distorted so that the origin of the pulmonary artery is displaced posteriorly and more rightward, whereas the origin of the aorta is displaced anteriorly and

Fig. 13–4. – Horizontal sections of hearts showing the great vessel relationship to the ventricles. Panel **A**, normal. Panel **B**, corrected transposition of the great arteries. Note that although in panel **B** the great vessels are transposed, the pulmonary artery continues to arise from the venous ventricle and the aorta from the arterial ventricle.

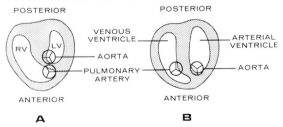

more leftward. Despite the displacement of the great arteries, the pulmonary artery continues to arise from the venous ventricle and the aorta from the arterial ventricle (Figs. 13–3 and 13–4).

The right and left branches of the conduction system remain with the appropriate anatomic ventricles. Since the ventricles are reversed in a right-to-left fashion, the position of the conduction system is similarly reversed. In the normal, the interventricular septum depolarizes from the side of the anatomic left ventricle toward the side of the anatomic right ventricle. Since in corrected transposition of the great arteries there is a reversal of the position of the anatomic ventricles as well as the conduction system, and since the interventricular septum continues to depolarize from the side of the anatomic left ventricle toward the side of the anatomic right ventricle, it should be apparent that, in the patient, the interventricular septum effectively depolarizes from right to left—a reversal of normal. In addition, this abnormal rotation can elongate the bundle of His to such a degree as to result in disruption of its fibers, causing complete heart block.

HEMODYNAMICS

In the absence of any intracardiac defects, the circulation is normal. Venous return is delivered to an anatomic right atrium, from which it passes through a two-leaflet mitral valve into an anatomic left ventricle. It leaves via the pulmonary artery (despite its displacement) into the lungs. Appropriately oxygenated blood returns into an anatomic left atrium, through a three-leaflet tricuspid valve and into an anatomic right ventricle. It finally leaves via the aorta (despite its displacement) and out the systemic circuit. Therefore, the patient with corrected transposition of the great arteries without intracardiac defects will have a normally functioning heart and may well go unrecognized as having congenital heart disease. However, there are clues to the diagnosis, and these will be elaborated on. The basic concept of corrected transposition of the great arteries can be characterized in the mnemonic

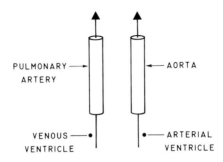

PULMONARY ARTERY

AORTA

VENOUS VENTRICLE

ARTERIAL VENTRICLE

The arrows represent blood flowing from the venous ventricle into the displaced pulmonary artery and from the arterial ventricle into the displaced aorta. If the blood flow is followed with the mnemonic in mind, the effect on the various chambers and vessels of the heart can be demonstrated by the following diagram:

RIGHT ATRIUM →
VENOUS VENTRICLE →
MAIN PULMONARY ARTERY →
PULMONARY VESSELS →

LEFT ATRIUM →
ARTERIAL VENTRICLE →
AORTA →

Fig. 13–5.—Chest roentgenograms of a child with corrected transposition of the great arteries demonstrating the straight upper left border of the heart representing the ascending aorta (*arrow* in the panel to the left and *dotted line* in the panel to the right). (Courtesy of P. Taber, M.D.)

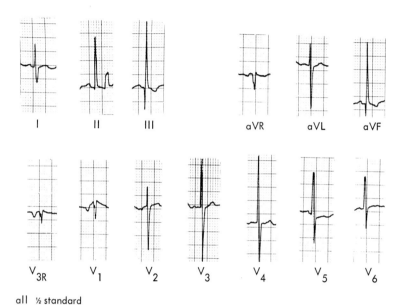

I	II	III	aVR	aVL	aVF

V$_{3R}$	V$_1$	V$_2$	V$_3$	V$_4$	V$_5$	V$_6$

all ½ standard

Fig. 13–6. – Electrocardiogram of a patient with corrected transposition of the great arteries, which demonstrates the presence of a Q in V$_6$.

The arrows represent alteration in the size of a chamber or a vessel as follows:

→ Unchanged

Translated to the chest x-ray, one would expect to find a heart normal in over-all size but with a peculiar configuration. The aorta dominates the upper left border of the heart, giving rise to an almost straight-line edge to that border (Fig. 13–5). Since there is no abnormality in chamber size, the electrocardiogram would be expected to be normal. However, because of the abnormalities in the conduction system noted above, it usually is not. Two findings are commonly seen. The first is the presence of a Q wave in leads III, aVF and V$_1$ and the absence of a Q wave in leads V$_5$ and V$_6$ (Fig. 13–6). The second is the presence of complete heart block (Fig. 13–7). Despite the logic in

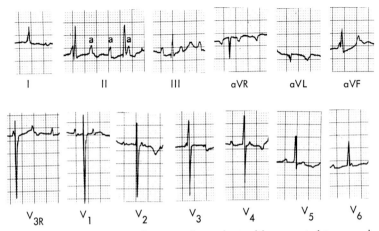

Fig. 13–7.—Electrocardiogram of a patient with corrected transposition of the great arteries showing complete heart block. The salient feature is the complete dissociation between the atria and the ventricles. a = P waves.

this situation, for reasons that are quite unclear, these electrocardiographic findings are not seen in all patients.

CLINICAL APPLICATION

As has been stated, the patient without a coexisting intracardiac defect can be totally missed and lead a normal life. This is the exception rather than the rule. It is much more common that the patient with corrected transposition of the great arteries has with it a ventricular septal defect with pulmonary hypertension, an Ebstein-like anomaly of the left atrioventricular valve (the tricuspid valve), pulmonary stenosis or, less commonly, any other intracardiac defect. Since the clinical picture is the result of the intracardiac defect and not of the transposed great arteries, a recitation of those findings would be redundant. Therefore, the reader is referred to the appropriate chapters for review, remembering that the basic malposition of the great arteries exists.

DIFFERENTIAL DIAGNOSIS

The patient with corrected transposition of the great arteries and associated defects must be differentiated from one having the same intracardiac defects but with normally positioned great arteries. If complete heart block or the abnormal Q wave distribution in the electrocardiogram or typical chest x-ray findings are present, the true diagnosis can be suspected. In the absence of these, however, cardiac catheterization will be required to establish the diagnosis.

PEARLS

1. This defect is more common in males than in females.

2. Coexisting intracardiac defects are the rule rather than the exception.

3. A ventricular septal defect with pulmonary hypertension is the most common lesion seen.

CHAPTER FOURTEEN

Total Anomalous Pulmonary Venous Connection

EMBRYOLOGY

AT ABOUT the third week of gestation, the pulmonary venous drainage develops. The lung buds are in communication with the splanchnic plexus, which, in turn, is connected to the umbilical vitelline veins and the cardinal veins (Fig. 14–1, *A*). At the same time, in the common atrium, there is an outpouching of a structure known as the common pulmonary vein, which grows to join the splanchnic plexus (Fig. 14–1, *B*). The cardinal veins and the umbilical vitelline veins then lose their connections with the splanchnic plexus. This leaves the pulmonary veins draining into the left atrium through the common pulmonary vein (Fig. 14–1, *C*). There is gradual absorption of the common pulmonary vein into the body of the left atrium, leading to the expected final relationship of four pulmonary veins draining into the left atrium proper (Fig. 14–1, *D*).

ANATOMY

Any disruption of this mechanism will result in an obligatory circuitous pathway from the common pulmonary vein to the heart. Four anomalous pathways are commonly seen. The first is from the common pulmonary vein through a vertical vein into the innominate vein to the right superior vena cava and into the right atrium (Fig. 14–2, *A*). The second is from the common pulmonary vein into the coronary sinus and then to the right

Fig. 14–1. – Diagrammatic representation of the embryologic development of the pulmonary venous drainage. Panels **A–D** show various stages of development. (See text for explanation.) *UV VEINS* = umbilical vitelline veins, *A* = common atrium, *CPV* = common pulmonary vein, *LA* = left atrium.

atrium (Fig. 14–2, *B*). The third is direct drainage into the right atrium as the result of absorption of the common pulmonary vein as four distinct pulmonary veins into that atrium (Fig. 14–2, *C*). The fourth is from the common pulmonary vein inferiorly into the portal vein, which reaches the right atrium via the ductus venosus and the inferior vena cava (Fig. 14–2, *D*).

Each of these communications can occur without any obstruction along the pulmonary venous pathway and be classified as total anomalous pulmonary venous connection without obstruction. Each of the communications can occur with obstruction along the pulmonary venous pathway and be classified as total anomalous pulmonary venous connection with obstruction. The presence or absence of obstruction so affects the entire clinical picture that separation into the two major classifications for further discussion is prudent at this point.

Fig. 14–2. – Diagrammatic representation of the anatomic variations of total anomalous pulmonary venous connection. (See text for explanation.) *SVC* = superior vena cava, *IVC* = inferior vena cava, *RA* = right atrium, *CS* = coronary sinus, *RV* = right ventricle, *LA* = left atrium, *LV* = left ventricle, *CPV* = common pulmonary vein, *VV* = vertical vein, *LPV* = left pulmonary veins, *RPV* = right pulmonary veins, *PV* = portal vein, *DV* = ductus venosus.

TOTAL ANOMALOUS PULMONARY VENOUS CONNECTION WITH OBSTRUCTION

Hemodynamics

The obstruction in the pulmonary venous channel raises the pulmonary venous pressure, causes the pulmonary vascular resistance to rise and results in pulmonary artery hypertension, placing a further pressure burden on the right ventricle. Pulmonary edema may result from the severe increase in pulmonary vascular pressure. This concept is demonstrated in the mnemonic

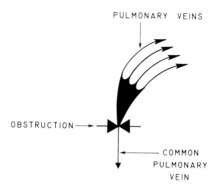

The single downward-pointing arrow being compressed by two horizontal arrows represents the obstruction of blood flow through the pulmonary vein. The multiple larger arrows pointing superiorly represent the backward pressure into the pulmonary veins. If the mnemonic is kept in mind, the effect on the heart can be demonstrated by the following diagram:

RIGHT ATRIUM →   LEFT ATRIUM →
RIGHT VENTRICLE →   LEFT VENTRICLE →
MAIN PULMONARY ARTERY →   AORTA →
PULMONARY VENOUS VESSELS ↑

The arrows represent alteration in the size of a chamber or a vessel as follows:

→ Unchanged
↑ Increased

This information can be translated to the chest x-ray, where one would expect to find a normal right atrium, a slightly enlarged right ventricle, a normal main pulmonary artery and increased pulmonary venous markings. The left atrium and left ventricle would be small. The over-all size of the heart is notably normal (Fig. 14–3). The electrocardiogram would show right ventricular hypertrophy (Fig. 14–4).

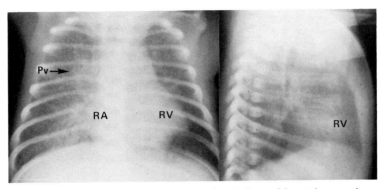

Fig. 14—3.—Chest roentgenograms of an infant with total anomalous pulmonary venous drainage with obstruction. Note the over-all small size of the heart and the punctate markings in the lungs representing pulmonary venous engorgement. RA = right atrium, RV = right ventricle, Pv = pulmonary venous engorgement.

Clinical Application

The clinical picture in such a patient is dependent on two sets of circumstances. The first is the amount of blood passing through the obstruction and where it goes, and the second, in an almost parenthetical sense, is the amount of blood that is unable to pass through the obstruction and where it goes.

Progressing forward first, the totally oxygenated blood that passes through the obstruction mixes with the venous blood returning from the superior and inferior venae cavae. The right atrial sample, therefore, will represent total venous mixing. The atrial septum is consistently patent, generally due to an anatomic atrial septal defect. As such, both the left atrium and the right ventricle will receive blood of equal saturation. Blood with the same degree of desaturation then will pass into the left ventricle and out the aorta, resulting in visible cyanosis. Since the volume of blood presented to the right atrium is relatively small, little turbulence will be created by passage of that blood across the tricuspid valve in diastole or out the pulmonary valve in systole. Therefore, murmurs may be nonexistent. In addition, right ventricular ejection time would not

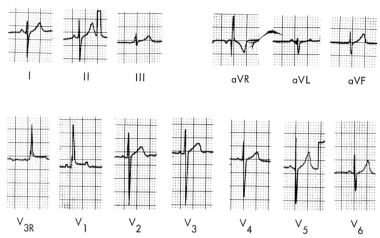

I   II   III   aVR   aVL   aVF

V_{3R} V_1 V_2 V_3 V_4 V_5 V_6

Fig. 14–4.—Electrocardiogram of an infant with total anomalous pulmonary venous drainage with obstruction. The salient feature is the dominant S_I and R_{III}—right axis deviation. There also is a dominant R wave in V_1 and S wave in $V_{5, 6}$, which is interpretable as right ventricular hypertrophy. The T wave in V_1 is also upright.

be prolonged and the second sound would not be widely split.

That blood unable to pass through the obstruction will be collected in the pulmonary venous system and may cause pulmonary edema. Marked tachypnea and dyspnea will result. With time, secondary right ventricular hypertrophy and right heart failure will become apparent.

Depending on the degree of obstruction, these events will become known in the first day to the first week of life. The diagnosis can be suspected in an infant of average size—usually a male—who has minimal cyanosis, minimal or no murmurs, marked tachypnea and dyspnea and possibly right heart failure. The electrocardiogram would show right ventricular hypertrophy and the chest x-ray would show a relatively normal sized heart but with increased pulmonary venous markings. The diagnosis can be confirmed with cardiac catheterization, during which one would expect to find comparable diminished oxygen saturations in each chamber and great artery, consistently elevated right ventricular pressures and commonly elevated right atrial pressures. A localized increase in oxygen saturation will mark the entrance of the anomalous vein (Table 14–1). Ideally, cineangiocardiography will demonstrate the course of the anomalous vessel.

As was stated earlier, obstruction to the common pulmonary vein can occur whether its insertion is below the diaphragm into the inferior vena cava or portal system or above the diaphragm into the innominate vein. In the former instance, the obstruction can be due to mechanical constriction of the vein as it passes through the diaphragm or to physiologic obstruction of flow as it passes through the ductus venosus and the liver. When the insertion is above the diaphragm, the obstruction generally is mechanical and due to passage of the vessel between any two fixed structures. When obstruction is present, regardless of the course of the vein, the physiologic events are the same.

TABLE 14–1.—IDEALIZED CARDIAC CATHETERIZATION DATA
IN A NEWBORN WITH TOTAL ANOMALOUS VENOUS CONNECTION
BELOW THE DIAPHRAGM*

SITE	PRESSURE (mm Hg)		OXYGEN SATURATION (%)	
	Normal	Patient	Normal	Patient
Common pulmonary vein			97	97
Superior vena cava			70	45
Inferior vena cava			74	70
Right atrium	a = 5 v = 3 m = 4	a = 10 v = 7 m = 8	72	55
Right ventricle	60/2	60/2	72	55
Main pulmonary artery	60/2	60/2	72	55
Left atrium	a = 5 v = 7 m = 6	a = 4 v = 6 m = 5	97	55
Left ventricle	60/2	60/2	97	55
Systemic artery	60/40	60/40	97	55

*The salient feature is an increase in oxygen saturation at the level of the inferior vena cava with final mixing in the right atrium. All other intracardiac values are identical. The pressures in the right atrium are elevated and those in the right ventricle and main pulmonary artery are systemic in height. The elevated pressures in the right side of the heart, in the normal, are a reflection of the expected fetal pulmonary hypertension seen in the newborn.

Differential Diagnosis

The patient with total anomalous pulmonary venous connection with obstruction must be differentiated from a patient having any other lesion causing cyanosis in infancy. This includes transposition of the great arteries, tricuspid atresia, truncus arteriosus and tetralogy of Fallot.

The patient with transposition of the great arteries may be confusing at the outset of the examination. However, the increase in pulmonary vascular markings will be arterial in nature, the heart will be enlarged and the mediastinum will be narrow. Since, in the first days of life, these findings will not be so obvious, cardiac catheterization generally will be necessary to make the differential.

The patient with tricuspid atresia will be eliminated in the differential when it is apparent that the electrocardiogram indicates left axis deviation and left ventricular hypertrophy.

The patient with tetralogy of Fallot rarely presents in the newborn period but, if so, the presence of markedly diminished pulmonary vascular markings assists in the differential.

The patient with truncus arteriosus also will be confusing at the outset of the examination but the chest x-ray will tend to show a somewhat enlarged heart with increased vascular markings. The presence of a systolic or a continuous murmur will be an additional aid. Cardiac catheterization will permit an accurate diagnosis.

TOTAL ANOMALOUS PULMONARY VENOUS CONNECTION WITHOUT OBSTRUCTION

When obstruction of the common pulmonary vein is not present, it is most likely that the insertion of that vein is above the diaphragm. Theoretically, it is possible for the common vein to empty below the diaphragm without obstruction and, if so, the physical findings would be no different. However, this is most uncommon, and so the remainder of this section will deal with the events that follow the anomalous connection of the pulmonary venous drainage above the diaphragm into the innominate vein. The basic challenge to the heart is that of increased flow to the right atrium, and is depicted in the mnemonic

If the blood flow is followed with the mnemonic in mind, the effect on the various chambers and vessels can be demonstrated by the following diagram:

MEDIASTINUM ↑   PULMONARY VESSELS ↑
RIGHT ATRIUM ↑   LEFT ATRIUM → ↓
RIGHT VENTRICLE ↑   LEFT VENTRICLE → ↓
MAIN PULMONARY ARTERY ↑   AORTA →

The arrows represent alteration in the size of a chamber or a vessel as follows:

→ Unchanged
↑ Increased
↓ Decreased

This information can be translated to the chest x-ray, where one would expect an enlarged right atrium, right ventricle and main pulmonary artery and increased pulmonary vascular markings. The left atrium would be small and the left ventricle small to normal. With time, the common pulmonary vein, which generally courses superiorly along the left side of the mediastinum, and the superior vena cava, which courses inferiorly along the right side of the mediastinum, will cause it to be wide and to give the appearance of a figure-of-eight or a snowman. This observation generally is not made until childhood (Fig. 14–5). The elec-

Fig. 14−5.−Chest roentgenograms of a child with total anomalous pulmonary venous drainage above the diaphragm without obstruction. Note the increase in cardiac size with the prominent right atrium and increase in pulmonary vascular markings. The mediastinum is also wide due to the anomalous drainage and resembles a figure-of-eight or a snowman. *RA* = right atrium, *RV* = right ventricle, *AV* = anomalous vessels, *PV* = pulmonary vessels.

trocardiogram would show right ventricular hypertrophy and, at times, right atrial hypertrophy (see Fig. 14−4).

Clinical Application

The patient with total anomalous pulmonary venous connection without obstruction generally is asymptomatic in infancy. In fact, the entire clinical picture is quite reminiscent of that due to an atrial septal defect. The entire pulmonary venous blood flow passes from the common pulmonary vein into the vertical vein and courses across to the superior vena cava. At each of these junctures, the systolic and diastolic flow can be heard as a high-pitched continuous murmur reminiscent of a venous hum (this is an uncommon finding). The pulmonary venous flow then augments the systemic venous return, delivering an extraordinary volume to the right atrium. Because of the obligatory interatrial communication, blood will flow both into the left atrium and across the tricuspid valve. The blood that passes across the valve may be heard as a mid-diastolic murmur. Right ventricular volume is increased and right ventricular systolic ejection time is prolonged. The passage of blood across the pulmonary valve will be heard as an ejection systolic murmur varying in intensity from grade II to grade III, medium in pitch and transmitting along the course of the pulmonary arterial vessels. The prolonged right ventricular ejection time will delay the closure of the pulmonary valve, resulting in a widely split second sound. The right ventricular volume overload is rather independent of venous return, and therefore fixed splitting of the second sound can be anticipated. The volume overload on the right side of the heart, which causes the right ventricular enlargement, will be palpable as a lift along the left sternal border.

The blood that passes into the left atrium remains desaturated (remember that the entire pulmonary venous return has already mixed with the systemic venous return) and the mixture eventually enters the aorta, accounting for the cyanosis generally seen.

The patient with total anomalous pulmonary venous connection is at risk for the early development of pulmonary vascular disease. Its presence will be suggested by a progressive narrowing of the splitting of the second sound, an increase in intensity of the pulmonary component and diminishing murmurs.

The diagnosis can be suspected in a patient — either male or female — who has relatively poor growth and development, a prominent left chest, a right ventricular heave, a systolic ejection murmur high along the left chest, a mild diastolic murmur low along the left chest and a widely split second sound. A chest x-ray showing enlargement of the right atrium and ventricle and increased pulmonary vascular markings should raise the possibility of a left-to-right shunt. The presence of the snowman configuration should significantly point to the proper diagnosis. In the presence of visible cyanosis, the picture becomes complete. The electrocardiogram should lend support if it shows right ventricular hypertrophy. The diagnosis can be finally confirmed with cardiac catheterization, during which one would find an increase in oxygen saturation in the superior vena cava, with identical oxygen saturations being present in all four intracardiac

TABLE 14–2.—IDEALIZED CARDIAC CATHETERIZATION DATA
IN A YOUNG CHILD WITH TOTAL ANOMALOUS PULMONARY
VENOUS DRAINAGE ABOVE THE DIAPHRAGM*

SITE	PRESSURE (mm Hg)		OXYGEN SATURATION (%)	
	Normal	Patient	Normal	Patient
Common pulmonary vein			97	97
Superior vena cava			70	88
Inferior vena cava			74	60
Right atrium	a = 5 v = 3 m = 4	a = 10 v = 7 m = 8	72	80
Right ventricle	25/2	40/2	72	80
Main pulmonary artery	25/12	40/12	72	80
Left atrium	a = 5 v = 7 m = 6	a = 4 v = 6 m = 5	97	80
Left ventricle	100/2	100/2	97	80
Systemic artery	100/60	100/60	97	80

*The salient feature is an oxygen saturation in the superior vena cava that is greater than that in the inferior vena cava. There is final mixing, with relative desaturation in the right atrium and identical values in all other chambers and both great arteries. The pressures in the right atrium are elevated, as are those in the right ventricle and the main pulmonary artery.

chambers as well as in both great arteries (Table 14–2). Cineangiocardiography would demonstrate the absence of any pulmonary venous connection directly to the left atrium and might well actually show the anomalous vessel.

Differential Diagnosis

The patient with total anomalous pulmonary venous connection without obstruction must be differentiated from one having a large atrial septal defect, a ventricular septal defect, truncus arteriosus and an atrioventricular canal.

The patient with an atrial septal defect will have similar clinical findings but will not be cyanotic either visibly or chemically. The presence of a wide mediastinum on x-ray will aid in the differential.

If the patient with a ventricular septal defect has a classic grade IV/VI holosystolic murmur, the differential will be easy.

If the patient has the Eisenmenger complex, peripheral desaturation will lend a note of confusion, but the absence of a snowman appearance on the heart will be helpful. Cardiac catheterization will permit an accurate differential.

The patient with a truncus arteriosus will be the most confusing in that the mediastinum may be wide and peripheral desaturation is consistently present. However, a single second sound will virtually establish the correct diagnosis. If necessary, cardiac catheterization and cineangiocardiography can finalize the differential.

The patient with an atrioventricular canal will be confusing in that the clinical picture may be similar but the cardiac silhouette on x-ray will be significantly greater and the electrocardiogram will show abnormal left axis deviation and biventricular hypertrophy. If necessary, cardiac catheterization can finalize the differential.

PEARLS

1. Patients with obstruction tend to be males whereas those without obstruction may be of either sex.

2. Total anomalous pulmonary venous connection with obstruction is virtually the only entity that gives congestive heart failure with a small heart.

3. The peripheral arterial desaturation that is consistently present without obstruction may be of such a minor degree as to make the presence of cyanosis difficult to ascertain.

CHAPTER FIFTEEN
Hypoplastic Left Heart Syndrome

EMBRYOLOGY

AT ABOUT the fifth week of gestation there is a blending of the anterior endocardial cushion, the posterior endocardial cushion, a portion of the interventricular septum and the ventricular muscle itself to form the left atrioventricular canal and subsequently the valve, known as the mitral valve (Figs. 15–1 and 15–2). The papillary muscles and chordae tendineae arise from the careful sculpturing of the ventricular muscle (Fig. 15–3). Slightly later, at about the sixth week of gestation, concomitant with the development of the truncus arteriosus, the aortic valve develops. It is formed by enlargement of three tubercles within the

Fig. 15–1. – Schematic representation of the common atrioventricular canal developing into a right and a left canal. **A,** 30 days; **B,** 33 days; **C,** 35 days. (See text for explanation.) (Modified from Moss, A. J., and Adams, F. H. [eds.]: *Heart Disease in Infants, Children and Adolescents* [Baltimore: The Williams & Wilkins Company, 1968], p. 17.)

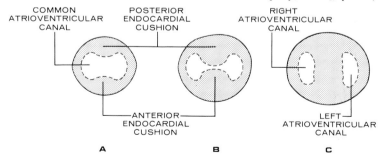

COMMON ATRIOVENTRICULAR CANAL   POSTERIOR ENDOCARDIAL CUSHION   RIGHT ATRIOVENTRICULAR CANAL

ANTERIOR ENDOCARDIAL CUSHION   LEFT ATRIOVENTRICULAR CANAL

A   B   C

157

Fig. 15–2.—Schematic representation of the formation of the mitral valve. (See text for explanation.) Identification of right-sided structures has been omitted intentionally. **A,** 37 days; **B,** newborn. (Modified from Moss, A. J., and Adams, F. H. [eds.]: *Heart Disease in Infants, Children and Adolescents* [Baltimore: The Williams & Wilkins Company, 1968], p. 16.)

lumen of the aorta, which grow toward the midline and finally are thinned by resorption of excess tissue. There is additional hollowing out of tissue at the superior portion of the tubercle at its junction with the wall of the aorta, giving rise to the sinuses of the valve (Figs. 15–4 and 15–5). At about the same time, the arches are differentiating, with the fourth arch destined to become the aorta (Fig. 15–6).

Fig. 15–3.—Schematic representation of the formation of the atrioventricular valves and their chordae tendineae and papillary muscles. (See text for explanation.) A and B, progressive stages of development. (Modified from Moss, A. J., and Adams, F. H. [eds.]: *Heart Disease in Infants, Children and Adolescents* [Baltimore: The Williams & Wilkins Company, 1968], p. 19.)

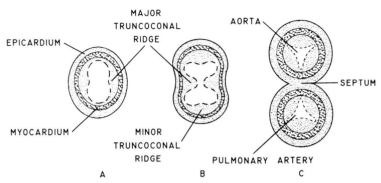

Fig. 15—4.—Schematic representation of the formation of the aortic valves within the aorta. Note the progressive proliferation of the trunco-conal ridges (the aortic valves are also demonstrated coincidentally). (Modified from Moss, A. J., and Adams, F. H. [eds.]: *Heart Disease in Infants, Children and Adolescents* [Baltimore: The Williams & Wilkins Company, 1968], p. 16.)

ANATOMY

If the mitral valve fails to develop totally, mitral atresia will result. If the aortic valve fails to develop totally, aortic atresia will result. If the arch of the aorta does not develop adequately, hypoplasia of the arch will result. Whether because of reduction of inflow due to mitral atresia or reduction of outflow due to aor-

Fig. 15—5.—A graphic demonstration of the proliferation and then hollowing out of the tubercles, giving rise to the completed valve.

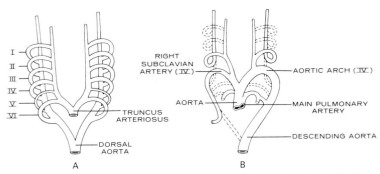

Fig. 15–6. — Diagrammatic representation of the embryologic development of the aortic arch system as it relates to the aorta. (See text for explanation.)

tic atresia or a hypoplastic arch, the common denominator is a diminutive left ventricular chamber (Fig. 15–7).

HEMODYNAMICS

It makes little difference whether the aortic valve or the mitral valve is atretic, either individually or in combination, for the dominant burden of both volume and pressure is placed on the

Fig. 15–7. — Diagrammatic representation of the anatomic appearance of a hypoplastic left heart. Note the diminutive left ventricle, a relatively small mitral valve and the very small aorta. RA = right atrium, RV = right ventricle, PA = pulmonary artery, LA = left atrium, LV = left ventricle.

right side of the heart. This concept is demonstrated in the mnemonic

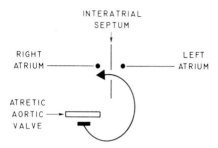

The heavy arrow represents the inability of blood to pass through the aortic valve, with resultant retrograde flow into the left atrium, through the interatrial septum and into the right atrium. The septum is demonstrated as a line and not a hole to suggest that the passage generally is through the foramen ovale and not through a true atrial septal defect. The same principle would apply if the obstruction were at the mitral valve (this is not demonstrated). If the flow of blood is followed with the mnemonic in mind, the effect on the various chambers and vessels of the heart can be demonstrated by the following diagram:

RIGHT ATRIUM ↑   LEFT ATRIUM ↓
RIGHT VENTRICLE ↑   LEFT VENTRICLE ↓
MAIN PULMONARY ARTERY ↑   AORTA ↓
PULMONARY VESSELS → ↑

The arrows represent alteration in the size of a chamber or a vessel as follows:

→ Unchanged
↑ Increased
↓ Decreased

Translated to the chest x-ray, one would expect to find cardiomegaly with right atrial, right ventricular and pulmonary artery enlargement. Also, the pulmonary vascularity might be increased. However, specific chamber enlargement frequently is

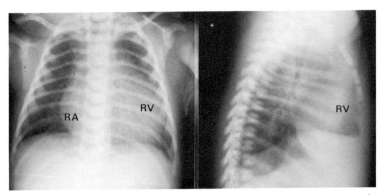

Fig. 15–8.—Chest roentgenograms of a newborn with hypoplastic left heart syndrome. Although there is a suggestion of an enlarged right atrium and right ventricle, the appearance basically is one of cardiomegaly. *RA* = right atrium, *RV* = right ventricle.

difficult to recognize in the newborn, and the chest x-ray may show only cardiomegaly (Fig. 15–8). The electrocardiogram would show right atrial and right ventricular hypertrophy with little or no left-sided forces (Fig. 15–9).

CLINICAL APPLICATION

It must be remembered that the patient with hypoplastic left heart syndrome is essentially living on blood flow from the right ventricle through the ductus arteriosus into the thoracic and descending aortae. The blood supply to the cerebral vessels and the coronary arteries is merely by retrograde flow. These circumstances place the baby in extreme jeopardy.

The infant may appear to be normal at birth, of average size and free from either cyanosis or pallor. Shortly thereafter, because of the obligatory intracardiac mixing, these signs will become apparent. The diminished retrograde hypoxemic coronary blood flow ultimately may lead to shock. The peripheral pulses will be small and the blood pressure, although equal throughout, will be low. The chest will be symmetric and a right ventricular heave palpable. The first sound will not be audibly unusual. The

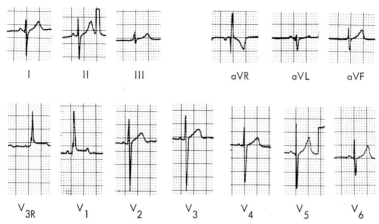

I II III aVR aVL aVF

V$_{3R}$ V$_1$ V$_2$ V$_3$ V$_4$ V$_5$ V$_6$

Fig. 15–9.—Electrocardiogram of a newborn with hypoplastic left heart syndrome. The salient feature is the dominant S$_I$ and R$_{III}$—right axis deviation. There also is a dominant R wave in V$_1$ and S wave in V$_{5, 6}$, which is interpretable as right ventricular hypertrophy. The T wave in V$_1$ is also upright.

second sound will be single, representing closure of only the pulmonary valve (a very important observation). The right ventricle acts as the systemic ventricle. Closure of the pulmonary valve becomes a function of systemic resistance and can be expected to be increased in absolute intensity. Generally, no murmur is heard.

The patient can be suspected of having hypoplastic left heart syndrome if he is newly born, in acute distress, with some cyanosis, pallor, poor peripheral pulses, a single second sound and no murmur. The presence of cardiomegaly and apparent right-sided enlargement on the chest x-ray along with an electrocardiogram that shows right ventricular hypertrophy and right atrial hypertrophy will strongly support the clinical impression. An echocardiogram can demonstrate a diminutive left ventricle, a poorly functioning or nonfunctioning mitral valve and a larger than normal right ventricle (Fig. 15–10). If doubt still exists, cardiac catheterization will define the lesion. The study will show an inability to enter or to demonstrate the left ventricle,

Fig. 15–10. — Echocardiograms in a normal newborn (**A**) and a patient with hypoplastic left heart syndrome (**B**). Note the very large right ventricle and very small left ventricle in the patient with hypoplastic left heart syndrome. *ECG* = electrocardiogram, *CW* = chest wall, *RV* = right ventricle, *S* = septum, *LV* = left ventricle, *MV* = mitral valve, *TV* = tricuspid valve. (Modified from Meyer, R. A., and Kaplan, S.: Prog. Cardiovasc. Dis. 15:341, 1973.)

some left-to-right shunting at the atrial level, systemic pressures in the right ventricle and the main pulmonary artery, normal to low pressures in the systemic artery and peripheral desaturation (Table 15–1).

DIFFERENTIAL DIAGNOSIS

If the patient with hypoplastic left heart syndrome is obviously cyanotic, he must be differentiated from one having any of the other major lesions causing cyanosis. These are transposition of the great arteries, tricuspid atresia, pulmonary atresia and, less commonly, truncus arteriosus, total anomalous pulmonary venous drainage and tetralogy of Fallot.

If the patient is basically pale rather than cyanotic, the differential should include consideration of abnormalities of the coronary arteries, such as anomalous origin of the left coronary artery from the pulmonary artery, calcification of the coronary arteries or, most rarely, thrombosis of a coronary vessel.

TABLE 15–1.—IDEALIZED CARDIAC CATHETERIZATION DATA IN A NEWBORN WITH HYPOPLASTIC LEFT HEART SYNDROME*

SITE	PRESSURE (mm Hg)		OXYGEN SATURATION (%)	
	Normal	Patient	Normal	Patient
Superior vena cava			70	60
Inferior vena cava			74	63
Right atrium	a = 5 v = 3 m = 4	a = 10 v = 8 m = 7	72	78
Right ventricle	60/5	60/5	72	78
Main pulmonary artery	60/30	60/30	72	78
Left atrium	a = 5 v = 7 m = 6	a = 15 v = 10 m = 10	97	97
Left ventricle	60/5	Not entered	97	Not entered
Systemic artery	60/45	60/40	97	78

*The salient features are an inability to enter the left ventricle and elevated pressures in the right ventricle and the pulmonary artery as well as both atria. There also is an increase in oxygen saturation in the right atrium and a decrease in the systemic artery.

PEARLS

1. The anomaly occurs more commonly in males than in females.

2. Early death is the rule.

3. The risk of cardiac catheterization in the newborn is 5% but should not deter one from performing the study when it is indicated.

4. With time, the echocardiogram may prove so effective in making the diagnosis as to obviate the need for cardiac catheterization.

5. Splitting of the second sound into two components rules out the diagnosis.

CHAPTER SIXTEEN
Endocardial Fibroelastosis

EMBRYOLOGY

FOR REASONS that are quite unclear, sometime during gestation the endocardium of the left atrium and the left ventricle becomes very thick. Although present at birth, endocardial fibroelastosis may not literally be a congenital defect but rather an intrauterine acquired insult. Implicated in the possible etiology are such things as intrauterine infection – either bacterial or viral – anoxia and nonspecific hereditary factors.

ANATOMY

The endocardial fibrotic thickening that is present can occur as a secondary phenomenon in the presence of coarctation of the aorta, aortic stenosis or other forms of hypoplastic left heart syndrome. It is also seen as an independent primary lesion classified into either a dilated or a contracted form. The more common dilated variety has a large left ventricular chamber with a thickened left ventricular wall. The endocardium is shiny and thick. The process may include the endocardium of the left atrium, the intervening mitral valve and its chordae tendineae, which, when involved, become foreshortened and/or the left ventricle.

The much less common contracted form has a small left ventricular chamber with a thickened left ventricular wall. The fibrotic process may well extend into the left atrium, the intervening mitral valve and its chordae tendineae. This is similar to the involvement in the dilated form.

This chapter will deal with the primary dilated form.

166

HEMODYNAMICS

The patient with endocardial fibroelastosis is confronted with a left ventricle that cannot contract normally. In the presence of marked elevation of the left ventricular end-diastolic pressure or mitral insufficiency, pulmonary hypertension can develop, leading to right ventricular hypertrophy. The basic left-sided events are depicted in the mnemonic

The black lining represents the thickened endocardium, which restricts normal contractility of the left ventricle. If the blood flow is followed with the mnemonic in mind, the effect on the heart can be demonstrated by the following diagram:

RIGHT ATRIUM →	LEFT ATRIUM → ↑
RIGHT VENTRICLE → ↑	LEFT VENTRICLE ↑
MAIN PULMONARY ARTERY → ↑	AORTA →
PULMONARY VESSELS →	

The arrows represent alteration in the size of a chamber or a vessel as follows:

→ Unchanged
↑ Increased

This information can be translated to the chest x-ray, where one would expect to find a normal right side, a normal or slightly enlarged left atrium and an enlarged left ventricle (Fig. 16–1). The electrocardiogram would consistently show left ventricular hypertrophy and possibly left atrial hypertrophy (Fig. 16–2). It is only very late in the clinical picture that right ventricular hy-

Fig. 16–1.—Chest roentgenograms of an infant with endocardial fibroelastosis. Note the gross cardiac enlargement, with depression of the apex due to left ventricular enlargement, and some enlargement of the right atrium and the right ventricle. *RA* = right atrium, *RV* = right ventricle, *LV* = left ventricle. (Courtesy of S. Sapin, M.D.)

pertrophy is seen in the electrocardiogram. This is not demonstrated.

CLINICAL APPLICATION

A patient with endocardial fibroelastosis will appear to be normal at birth and continue so for the first few months of life. To meet the increased metabolic demands occurring with growth, the heart will enlarge mainly at the expense of the left ventricle. It will continue to hypertrophy until it fails, at which time tachypnea, dyspnea, tachycardia and hepatomegaly – the symptoms and signs of congestive heart failure – will be seen. The resultant cardiomegaly will distort the left side of the chest. The apical impulse will be displaced laterally and inferiorly and the action of the left ventricle will be felt as a thrust. The first sound should be normal. The second sound should be normal also, being variably split with normal pulmonary and aortic components. The advent of pulmonary hypertension will be heralded by an increase in intensity of the pulmonary component of

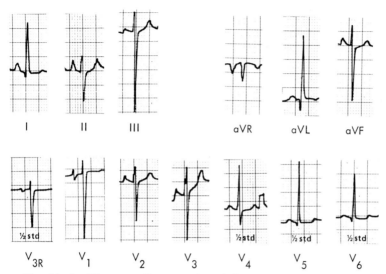

I II III aVR aVL aVF

½std

V_{3R} V_1 V_2 V_3 ½std V_4 ½std V_5 ½std V_6

Fig. 16–2.—Electrocardiogram of an infant with endocardial fibro-elastosis. The salient feature is a dominant R_I and S_{III}—left axis deviation. There also is a deep S wave in lead V_1 and a very tall R wave in leads $V_{5,\ 6}$, which is interpretable as left ventricular hypertrophy.

TABLE 16–1.—IDEALIZED CARDIAC CATHETERIZATION DATA
IN AN INFANT WITH ENDOCARDIAL FIBROELASTOSIS*

SITE	PRESSURE (mm Hg)		OXYGEN SATURATION (%)	
	Normal	Patient	Normal	Patient
Superior vena cava			70	70
Inferior vena cava			74	74
Right atrium	a = 5 v = 3 m = 4	a = 5 v = 3 m = 4	72	72
Right ventricle	25/2	35/2	72	72
Main pulmonary artery	25/2	35/15	72	72
Left atrium	a = 5 v = 7 m = 6	a = 13 v = 17 m = 16	97	97
Left ventricle	100/5	100/15	97	97
Systemic artery	100/75	100/75	97	97

*The salient feature is slight elevation of pressure in the right ventricle, main pulmonary artery and left atrium. There also is selective elevation of the diastolic pressure in the left ventricle. The oxygen saturations are normal.

A **B**

Fig. 16–3.—Enlargement of two frames from a 35-mm cineangio-cardiogram of a normal patient. Note the size of the left ventricle in diastole (**A**) as compared to systole (**B**). *C* = catheter, *LA* = left atrium, *LV* = left ventricle, *Ao* = aorta.

the second sound. Generally no murmur is heard. However, if mitral insufficiency is present, it will be recognized by a high-pitched holosystolic murmur, loudest at the apex with transmission into the left axilla.

Therefore, the diagnosis of endocardial fibroelastosis can be suspected in a patient—usually under 6 months of age—who has

Fig. 16–4.—Enlargement of two frames from a 35-mm cineangio-cardiogram of a patient with endocardial fibroelastosis. Note the very little difference in size of the left ventricle in diastole (**A**) as compared to systole (**B**). *C* = catheter, *LA* = left atrium, *LV* = left ventricle, *Ao* = aorta.

A **B**

congestive heart failure, no murmur, gross cardiomegaly both on physical examination and in the chest x-ray and left ventricular hypertrophy in the electrocardiogram. It can be confirmed by cardiac catheterization, during which one would find normal to elevated right ventricular pressure, elevated left ventricular end-diastolic pressure, no intracardiac shunts and restricted motion of the left ventricle as viewed in angiocardiography (Table 16–1 and Figs. 16–3 and 16–4).

DIFFERENTIAL DIAGNOSIS

The patient with primary endocardial fibroelastosis must be differentiated from a patient with anomalous origin of the left coronary artery, glycogen storage disease of the heart, calcification of the coronary arteries, myocarditis, pericarditis with effusion and supraventricular tachycardia with congestive heart failure.

The patient with anomalous left coronary artery is similar in general appearance and physical findings. However, the electrocardiogram consistently shows an abnormal Q wave in leads I, aVL and V_5 or V_6. These observations are very reminiscent of the adult with an anterior myocardial infarction.

Patients with glycogen storage disease of the heart are quite difficult to distinguish. However, they rarely live beyond 3–6 months of age, which is about the time that patients with endocardial fibroelastosis most commonly begin having difficulty.

Calcification of the coronary arteries is an extremely rare condition. It would mimic an anomalous left coronary artery in that the obstruction to coronary flow might result in an infarct pattern. Cardiac fluoroscopy may reveal the calcification.

The patient with myocarditis may be very confusing, but the history and general appearance of an overwhelming systemic illness as well as the cardiac involvement should be a clue.

Recognition of pericardial effusion is extraordinarily important, for restriction of normal contractility is exterior to the heart and treatable by pericardiocentesis. There would be no evidence of left ventricular hypertrophy on the electrocardiogram. An echocardiogram would be of maximal help in identifying the pericardial fluid. Other radiographic techniques are available also.

The patient with supraventricular tachycardia with congestive heart failure should be recognized promptly on the basis of the heart rate and the electrocardiogram.

PEARLS

1. Remember that this group of patients presents with quite similar clinical pictures but that endocardial fibroelastosis is the most common lesion.

2. There is a significant familial incidence.

BIBLIOGRAPHY

Edwards, J. E., Carey, L. S., Neufeld, H. N., and Lester, R. G.: *Congenital Heart Disease.* Correlation of Pathologic Anatomy and Angiocardiography (Philadelphia and London: W. B. Saunders Company, 1965), 2 vols.

Fontana, R. S., and Edwards, J. E.: *Congenital Cardiac Disease.* A Review of 357 Cases Studied Pathologically (Philadelphia and London: W. B. Saunders Company, 1962).

Gasul, B. M., Arcilla, R. A., and Lev, M.: *Heart Disease in Children* (Philadelphia and Montreal: J. B. Lippincott Company, 1966).

Keith, J. D., Rowe, R., and Ulad, P.: *Heart Disease in Infancy & Childhood* (2d ed.; New York: The Macmillan Company, 1967).

Kirklin, J. W., and Karp, R. B.: *The Tetralogy of Fallot.* From a Surgical Viewpoint (Philadelphia, London and Toronto: W. B. Saunders Company, 1970).

Kjellberg, S. R., Mannheimer, E., Rudhe, U., and Jonsson, B.: *Diagnosis of Congenital Heart Disease* (2d ed.; Chicago: Year Book Medical Publishers, Inc., 1959).

Krovitz, L. J., Gessner, I. H., and Scheibler, G. L.: *Handbook of Pediatric Cardiology* (New York: Hoeber Medical Division, Harper & Row, Publishers, 1969).

Moss, A. J., and Adams, F. H. (eds.): *Heart Disease in Infants,*

Children and Adolescents (Baltimore: The Williams & Wilkins Company, 1968).

Nadas, A. S., and Fyler, D. C.: *Pediatric Cardiology* (3d ed.; Philadelphia, London and Toronto, 1972).

Perloff, J. K.: *The Clinical Recognition of Congenital Heart Disease* (Philadelphia, London and Toronto: W. B. Saunders Company, 1970).

Rowe, R. D., and Mehrizi, A.: *The Neonate with Congenital Heart Disease* (Philadelphia, London and Toronto: W. B. Saunders Company, 1968).

Taussig, H. B.: *Congenital Malformations of the Heart* (Cambridge, Mass.: Published for The Commonwealth Fund by Harvard University Press, 1960), 2 vols.

Venables, A. W.: *Essentials of Pediatric Cardiology* (Springfield, Ill.: Charles C Thomas, Publisher, 1964).

Index

type II, 118
type IV, 120
Roentgenography (*see*
   Radiography)

S

Septal defect
  atrial, 1 – 8
    anatomy, 2 – 3
    cardiac catheterization in,
      idealized, 6
    clinical application, 5 – 6
    diagnosis, differential, 7
    embryology, 1 – 2
    hemodynamics, 3 – 5
    ostium primum type, 6 – 7
    ostium primum type, ECG
      of, 7
    ostium secundum type, ECG
      of, 4
    pearls, 8
    radiography of, 4
    types, schematic
      representation of, 2
  ventricular, 9 – 24
    anatomy, 10 – 11
    classic, 12 – 15
    classic, catheterization in,
      idealized cardiac, 14
    classic, clinical application,
      14 – 15
    classic, ECG of, 13
    classic, hemodynamics, 12 –
      14
    classic, radiography of, 13
    diagnosis, differential, 23
    embryology, 9 – 10
    hemodynamics, 11 – 12
    natural history, 21 – 22
    pearls, 23 – 24
    small, 15 – 16
    small, clinical application,
      15 – 16
    small, hemodynamics, 15

supracristal, 16
transposition and (*see*
   Transposition of great
   arteries, with ventricular
   septal defect)
Septum
  interatrial, formation of, 1, 34
  interventricular (*see*
    Interventricular septum)
  ventricular, final fusion of, 116
Shunt, left ventricle to right
   atrial, 20 – 21
  clinical application, 21
  hemodynamics, 20 – 21
Sounds: in pulmonary stenosis,
   61
Stenosis
  aortic, 42 – 54
    (*See also* subaortic *below*)
    anatomy, 44
    diagnosis, differential, 54
    embryology, 42 – 44
    pearls, 54
    subvalvular, discrete, 52 – 53
    supravalvular, 53 – 54
  aortic, valvular, 44 – 49
    catheterization in, idealized
      cardiac, 48 – 49
    clinical application, 45 – 49
    ECG of, 46
    hemodynamics, 44 – 45
    radiography of, 46
  infundibular, 63 – 64
  pulmonary, 55 – 67
    anatomy, 56 – 57
    artery, peripheral, 64 – 66
    artery, peripheral,
      classification of, 65
    clinical application, 59 – 66
    diagnosis, differential, 66
    ejection click in, 61
    hemodynamics, 57 – 59
    malignant, 61 – 62
    pearls, 66 – 67
    sounds in, 61